REASONS AND EXPERIENCE

Reasons and Experience

ALAN MILLAR

CLARENDON PRESS · OXFORD
1991

Oxford University Press, Walton Street, Oxford OX2 6DP
Oxford New York Toronto
Dehli Bombay Calcutta Madras Karachi
Petaling Jaya Singapore Hong Kong Tokyo
Nairobi Dar es Salaam Cape Town
Melbourne Auckland
and associated companies in
Berlin Ibadan

Oxford is a trade mark of Oxford University Press

Published in the United States
by Oxford University Press, New York

British Library Cataloguing in Publication Data
Millar, Alan
Reasons and experience.
1. Philosophy
I. Title
100
ISBN 0-19-824270-0

Library of Congress Cataloging in Publication Data
Millar, Alan, Ph.D.
Reasons and experience/Alan Millar.
Includes bibliographical references and index.
1. Senses and sensation. 2. Philosophy of mind. 3. Knowledge, Theory of. 4. Belief and doubt. I. Title.
BD214.M49 1991 121'.3—dc20 90–45738
ISBN 0-19-824270-0

Set by Pentacor PLC, *High Wycombe, Bucks*
Printed and bound in Great Britain by
Biddles Ltd, Guildford and King's Lynn

For my parents,
Pearl and John Millar

Preface

Although little is said in this book about Kant there is no doubt that its main theme is Kantian for it concerns the relation between the intellect or understanding and the senses. It has long seemed to me that many modern discussions of this theme over-intellectualize the senses, treating the sensory experiences we typically have in perception as, in effect, propositional attitudes albeit of a peculiar sort. In this book I am critical of this general approach and develop an alternative view, following through its implications for the theory of knowledge. *En route* I have much to say about concepts, conceptual capacities, beliefs and the conditions under which beliefs are justified. The Introduction provides a synopsis of the entire discussion.

Throughout I have tried to provide as much analytical detail as seemed necessary to make my views plausible, while at the same time developing a broad perspective on the issues. I have also introduced historical considerations where these seemed to be of interest. Though I make use of a certain amount of jargon I do not presuppose a detailed knowledge of particular philosophical stances or technicalities. The book is aimed principally at professional philosophers, but I have sought to make it accessible to intermediate and advanced students of philosophy. I hope also that it may be of some interest to cognitive psychologists.

I am aware of a general debt to the writings of Wilfred Sellars which may well be greater than my footnotes indicate. Sellars's work seems to me to be among the most penetrating and thought-provoking to have been produced this century.

I am grateful to my philosophical colleagues at Stirling both for lively seminar discussions on material covered in this book and for their support and encouragement over many years. Regular discussions with Andrew Brennan and Tony Pitson have been invaluable. Antony Duff supplied me with written comments on early draft material which helped me to avoid errors. Discussions in undergraduate classes have forced me to clarify my views at crucial points. I have also benefited from discussion of early draft material at gatherings at the Universities of Aberdeen and St Andrews and at the Scots Philosophical Club meeting held at Stirling in December 1987. Thanks are due to Elspeth Gillespie for efficient and willing secretarial assistance. Above all, I owe an immense debt of gratitude to Rose-Mary and Stéphane Millar. Without their support, patience, and tolerance this book would not have been completed.

A number of passages in the book are drawn from articles of mine in print. I am grateful to the Aristotelian Society for permission to reproduce material in 'What's in a Look?' which appears in the Society's Proceedings for 1985/6, and to the Editor of *Ratio* for permission to reproduce material in 'Experience and the Justification of Belief' which appears in *Ratio*, 2, 1989.

A. M.
University of Stirling
September 1990

Contents

Introduction

This book deals with topics on the borderlands between the philosophy of mind and the theory of knowledge. My main concern is with sensory experiences and their role in relation to the justification of beliefs. Chapter 1 presents a fairly detailed treatment of sensory experience focusing on issues falling within what may be called the theory of the content of psychological states. Subsequent chapters deal with how our beliefs are justified and give special attention to the question of whether, and if so how, sensory experiences contribute to their justification.

It is a commonplace among many philosophers that sensory experiences, hereafter called simply experiences, have propositional contents. This way of thinking is made natural, among other things, by the fact that experiences may readily be described in terms of propositional clauses spelling out how things seem to the subject. It may seem to you that thunder is rumbling in the distance, that a coffee-stain is on the table-cloth, that the lamb you are eating is flavoured with rosemary, and so forth. In the light of this it is tempting to regard experiences as a kind of propositional attitude, to be regarded as having propositional content in the way that beliefs and desires do. I take it to be an implication of such a view that the content of an experience is intrinsic to the type of the experience, in the sense that any experience of the same type would have to have the same content. The burden of Chapter 1 is to argue that such a view is mistaken.

Crucial to the argument is the distinction between the notion of an experience's being *such that it seems to the subject that an F is there* and the notion of an experience's being *F-type*. An *F*-type experience is, roughly speaking, an experience of the type which an *F* would yield, that is, would produce under certain suitability and normality conditions. An experience is such that it seems to the subject that an *F* is there if it is such that in the absence of countervailing considerations its subject would believe that an *F* is there. Combining these two notions we may say that an experience is *of an F* if it is *F*-type and such that it seems to the subject that an *F* is there. (In place of '*F*' go predicates pertaining to things in the environment. It is a matter for debate what more precise restrictions should be placed on substituends for '*F*'.) I claim that different subjects may each have token experiences which are phenomenally identical in that each is *F*-type, say, and in all other respects the same, yet the experience of one subject is such that it seems to that subject that an *F* is there, while the experience of the other subject is such that it does not seem to that subject that an *F* is there. The possibility that this should be so brings out the sense in which the content that an *F* is there is not intrinsic to the experiences in question. The typology of experience which helps to make this plausible is set out in 1.4.

Throughout this book I write as if we can all agree that there are such things as experiences even if we differ over what account to give of them. I certainly hold that we should all be able to agree on this. Nothing seems less problematic than that when we perceive something we are in a conscious state which we could be in even if we were not perceiving that thing. These conscious states are what I call experiences. This much is accepted by philosophers who differ radically from me on what account to give of experiences. It is accepted, for instance, by those who think of experiences as something like inclinations to belief caused by sensory stimulation. Nevertheless, it is a fact that some philosophers do find talk of experiences puzzling, largely, I think, because of misconceptions about what such talk commits one to. It may help readers right at the start to take note of two views which are indeed open to objection, but to which I am not committed.

One view is that experiences are the 'immediate' objects of perception. Here the idea is that in so far as we perceive objects in the environment we do so via the perception of our own current experiences. The trouble is that we do not in any sense perceive our own experiences. What can be perceived can be surveyed from different points of view. Experiences cannot be surveyed and are not examined from a point of view. In perceiving our environment we have experiences, but these experiences are not intermediaries between us and the environment. The other view is that experiences are supposed to have a special epistemological role such that all our knowledge of the environment rests on knowledge of our own current experiences. This view is plausible only if the first view is plausible and is thus open to objection on that account. Unless experiences are immediate objects of perception there is little reason to suppose that our knowledge of the environment rests on knowledge of them. Still, the view is worth a special mention if only because it might seem to supply the primary motivation for the idea that we have experiences. In this book I am concerned with the epistemological role of experiences, but nothing in what follows implies that our knowledge of our current experiences is the foundation of our knowledge of the world about us.

The main discussion of the epistemological role of experiences occurs in Chapter 4, where I argue that experiences do not merely cause beliefs, but contribute to their justification. In dealing with questions about justification, many philosophers restrict themselves to the circle of beliefs. Experiences or stimulations enter the picture as causal determinants of beliefs rather than justifiers. This view has been explicitly proposed by Donald Davidson among others. In Chapter 4 I argue that experiences themselves contribute to the justification of beliefs about the world around us and that when they do other beliefs are always implicated. A belief about the environment never derives its justification from experience alone.

In Chapters 2 and 3 I develop an account of reasons and justification designed among other things to prepare the way for the discussion in Chapter 4. Chapter 2 has an account of derived justification according to which a subject's belief that *p* derives its justification from his beliefs that *q*, *r*, . . . only if (i) the belief that *p* is based, in a causal sense, on the beliefs *q*, *r*, . . .; (ii) there is a rational connection between the proposition that *p* and the propositions that *q*, *r*, . . .; (iii) the subject's basing his belief that *p* on his beliefs that *q*, *r*, . . . is an exercise of competence on his part with respect to the patterns of inference which underwrite the rational connection between the relevant propositions, and lastly, (iv) the subject legitimately takes for granted that *q*, *r*, ... Condition (ii) is fulfilled only if the propositions that *q*, *r*, . . . constitute what I call an *unconditional reason* for thinking that *p*. This will be true if the proposition that *p* may be inferred from the propositions that *q, r, . . .* without further ado. Unconditional reasons should not be conflated with conclusive reasons. In the sense intended here a set of propositions constitute a conclusive reason for some proposition if and only if it is impossible that the latter be false and the former true. Not all unconditional reasons are conclusive.

The concept of competence with respect to an inference pattern is of interest on at least two counts. There are imaginable cases in which a belief that *p* is based on others and (ii) satisfied, yet the fact that (ii) is satisfied has nothing to do with the subject's believing that *p*. In these cases it is accidental that the beliefs in question are rationally connected. Intuitively, when a belief is justified it should not be merely accidental that the contents of the beliefs on which it is based constitute an unconditional reason for the content of the belief in question. Condition (iii) rules out accidental rational connections. The other reason why the notion of competence is of interest is that it feeds into a plausible view of concepts. If, as a first approximation, we think of concepts as being individuated by patterns of inference, we may think of possessing a concept as a matter of being governed by those patterns. The relevant notion of governance is explored in 2.2.

The sorts of unconditional reasons which are my main concern in Chapters 2 and 3 are those implicated in basing beliefs on evidence, where the evidence is of a type which reliably, but not infallibly, indicates the occurrence of an event or state of affairs of some type. The reasons involved here are inconclusive. In 2.4 I discuss at some length a simple example in which we believe that deer have passed on seeing tracks of a certain sort on a path. In Chapter 3 this example is then used as a model to compare and contrast a type of case which has been thought to be philosophically problematic, namely that in which we believe that a person is in pain on the basis of beliefs about that person's behaviour. In both cases an evidential proposition is involved, that is, a proposition to the effect that *e* is evidence for *h*, but some philosophers have argued that pain behaviour is a criterion of pain. On this view, it is a necessary truth that, for instance, wincing is evidence of pain. I reject this view, but attempt to do justice to the thought that the status of a proposition such as that wincing is evidence of pain is different from the status of the proposition that the occurrence of tracks of a certain sort is evidence of the recent passage of deer. I propose that the former proposition is contingent yet normative in a sense which allows for the possibility that it may be legitimately taken for granted even in the absence of supporting grounds. In Chapter 3 the proposal is introduced and in Chapter 6 the idea that there are groundless yet legitimately held beliefs is further defended.

The discussion of Chapters 2 and 3 is independent of that of Chapter 1 in that it does not stand or fall with the views defended there. In Chapter 4 the themes of the first three chapters are pulled together. At that stage we have to hand an account of conditions which must be satisfied in cases where beliefs derive their justification from other beliefs. Call these doxastic cases. The governing thought of Chapter 4 is that we could make sense of there being experiential cases, that is, cases in which beliefs derive justification at least in part from the current experiences of the subject, if we can find plausible and suitable analogues for the conditions of justified belief which apply to doxastic cases. This project might seem to be hampered by the results of Chapter 1. If experiences are not intrinsically contentful then one might wonder how there could be plausible analogues for conditions (ii) and (iii) which apply to doxastic cases. The main thrust of Chapter 4 is that this prima-facie difficulty can be met with the help of the idea (1) that experience types have quasi-inferential links with propositions and (2) that some of our conceptual capacities are plausibly accounted for on the assumption that the concepts concerned are individuated in part by patterns of quasi-inference. As well as addressing the problem in hand the discussion extends the considerations about concepts begun in Chapter 2.

Much of the philosophical interest of Chapter 4 arises from the fact that it shows how beliefs can derive justification at least in part from the current experience of the subject while keeping to the spirit of the theory of justification for doxastic cases outlined in Chapters 2 and 3. The resulting extended theory of justification is regulative in so far as it implies that justified beliefs must be formed or sustained in a manner which depends on the fact that the subject is regulated by certain constraints.

The constraints are imposed by the relevant inference or quasi-inference patterns. The appropriateness or inappropriateness of the basis of a belief that *p* to the belief that *p* turns on these patterns. Beliefs about the present environment based on current experience might be thought to create a special difficulty for regulative theories. The thought would be that if we were guided by considerations pertaining to the appropriateness of experiences to beliefs we would consider our current experiences before forming beliefs on their basis. Yet clearly we do no such thing. The solution lies in an account of the relevant kinds of competence which, while requiring us to appreciate the appropriateness of experiences of such-and-such types to beliefs of such-and-such types, does not require consideration of current experiences when forming or sustaining beliefs on their basis.

Another important feature of the theory of justification is the role it gives to conceptual capacities. The competence which is exercised in the formation and maintenance of justified beliefs is competence in the mastery of concepts. Since epistemology is surely concerned with the examination of significant modes of justification it follows that a central task of epistemology must be to shed light on important classes of concepts and the capacities in which their mastery consists. This being so epistemology will have a close kinship with the theory of content and with semantics.

In Chapter 5 I contrast my *conceptualist* approach to epistemology with what I call *nativism*. Nativists seek an understanding of the constraints on justified belief through the scientific examination of native cognitive capacities like perception, memory, and concept acquisition. The programme requires a close *rapprochement* between epistemology and psychology. Indeed, Quine goes so far as to regard epistemology as a chapter of psychology. It is tempting to regard nativism as a new departure. I spend some time in Chapter 5 showing that Locke and Hume were nativists and that Quine and Goldman are very much in the classical tradition. This requires a fair amount of exegetical work which may not be to the taste of all readers. Nevertheless, these case-studies serve to illustrate nativism and thus to locate my own conceptualist approach in relation to past and present work. More importantly, perhaps, they illustrate a problem for nativism. The tendency of nativism is to give priority in the order of enquiry to native cognitive capacities. My worry here is a very simple one. Our conceptions of how our native cognitive capacities function in acquiring knowledge depends on an understanding of our conceptual capacities, an understanding which must be gleaned from reflection on how we form, maintain, and abandon beliefs and how we evaluate beliefs. In Chapter 5 I show that there are problems for the nativist approaches which I discuss which stem from a failure to appreciate this point. It is no part of my aim to show that epistemology is a purely a priori enterprise or to pour cold water on the idea that there is a significant overlap between the aims of philosophers and psychologists in this area. I am concerned to argue that progress in understanding our native cognitive capacities must be built on a conceptualist epistemology.

An important strand in my treatment of justification is that beliefs can be justificationally dependent on groundless beliefs. If the belief that *p* derives its justification from the beliefs that *q*, *r*, . . . then it must be legitimate for the subject to take for granted that *q*, *r*, ... Sometimes it is legitimate to take something for granted because one has adequate grounds for believing it. I argue that it can be legitimate to take something for granted even though one has no grounds for believing it. (I prefer to reserve the term 'justified' for beliefs held on grounds, that is, based on other beliefs or a complex of beliefs and experiences.) The main discussion of these matters occurs in Chapter 6. The chapter commences with a brief critique of foundationalist epistemology largely based on the claim that it is psychologically unrealistic. This serves to underline the fact that my own treatment of the justificatory role of experience is not motivated by foundationalism. It also advances my general epistemological approach since the critique of foundationalism testifies to the importance in our thinking of groundless beliefs which would not count as being legitimately held on any foundationalist view as normally conceived. This theme is developed further via a discussion of Wittgenstein's *On Certainty*. Drawing on hints provided by Wittgenstein I make use of the notion that certain propositions have a normative role in our thinking in that they are placed beyond doubt and dispute and their acceptance can be legitimate even in the absence of grounds. These propositions and the concepts we possess form our perspective on the world. In learning how to manage our own beliefs and evaluate beliefs generally we must acquire a mastery of a perspective. This means that we must learn not only how to employ concepts but how to make use of the propositions which are normative for us.

An obvious problem with any view which countenances legitimately held groundless beliefs is that it sanctions dogma and credulity. I argue that there are constraints relevant to when a groundless belief is legitimate which rule out both dogma and credulity. We may not hold on to a groundless belief in the face of a conflict between it and other beliefs for which we have adequate grounds. Nor may we accept any proposition we please in the absence of adequate grounds. In the course of the discussion I introduce the notion of an ideal rationality requirement. An example would be: Avoid accepting propositions which conflict with one another. I distinguish between such requirements and what is required for competence in mastering our perspective on the world. It turns out that competence does not require ideal rationality. Competence is the concept which figures in the conditions of justified belief. Beliefs may be justified yet held in breach of ideal rationality requirements.

The final chapter is a discussion of *scepticism*. After a brief treatment of the idea that we should suspend all our beliefs about the world around us the focus is on scepticism with regard to whether any of our beliefs are justified. Crude sceptical strategies posit various 'right' conditions on justified belief and argue that beliefs which by our ordinary standards are justified do not satisfy the right conditions. Such strategies, I claim, are undermined by the fact that the sceptic has no adequate rationale for his austere 'right' conditions. I then consider a sophisticated strategy which bases scepticism on a demand which is supposed to be written into our ordinary thinking about justification, rather than imposed arbitrarily by the sceptic. The demand is that modes of genuine justification be truth-indicative. The rationale for this demand is supposed to be found in the idea that we aim to believe only what is true. I agree that we aim to believe only what is true and that therefore we certainly want our modes of justification to be truth-indicative. It does not follow from this that genuine justification must be in a truth-indicative mode. Our justified beliefs are ones with respect to which, roughly speaking, we have done what we feasibly could to ensure that we believe only what is true. This leaves room for the possibility that some of our modes of justification are not truth-indicative. The upshot is that the sophisticated sceptic misunderstands what aiming at truth requires of us.

My primary concern in this book is with what we may legitimately believe. Traditionally, enquiries of this sort have been linked to very practical worries about what to think and how to proceed in thinking. Thus for the great epistemologists of the seventeenth and eighteenth centuries disputes about what may be believed and how best to achieve advances in knowledge had a direct bearing on method in what we now think of as the natural sciences, and a direct bearing on religious, ethical, and political convictions. The enquiry into human understanding was meant to disclose the nature of our cognitive capacities and how they may best function. It could thus be used to determine whether the pursuit of certain sorts of investigation or the holding of certain sorts of beliefs is consistent with the proper use of these capacities. Granted the role of variable perspectives in the formation and maintenance of beliefs it seems unlikely that an examination of shared cognitive capacities will provide the kind of general guide to enquiry and legitimate belief which the classical epistemologists sought. Yet epistemology conceived as in this book can make a difference to our practical reflections on what is worthy of belief. For one thing it can correct simplistic models of legitimate belief, for instance, models which assume that legitimate beliefs must be based on grounds. It can also alert us to the ever-present danger of a parochial use of 'we' in philosophy and ordinary life, the danger, that is to say, of taking what 'we' believe as constituting a world-picture demanding acceptance by all reasonable people.

1

Sensory Experience

1.1. *Sensations and Propositional Attitudes*

Sensory experiences are the sorts of experiences we have when we see, hear, touch, smell, or taste something. They provide topics both for the theory of knowledge and the philosophy of mind. The theory of knowledge is concerned with the way in which experiences yield knowledge of the world about us. Central to that enquiry is the question of how experiences warrant or justify beliefs. The philosophy of mind is concerned with experiences as a species of mental state. It considers what kind of mental state they are and how they relate to other mental states like beliefs and desires. It is this latter topic which I shall pursue in this chapter leaving epistemological matters, for the most part, to later chapters.

It is customary to draw a distinction between two kinds of mental state, *sensations* and *propositional attitudes*.[1] Sensations include itches, tickles, feelings of numbness, and experiences generally. Propositional attitudes are states like belief, desire, intention, and hope, in which the subject has an attitude to some proposition. Arguably, the central attitudes are belief and desire. Belief is the attitude of taking some proposition to be true. Thus, one who believes that the Prime Minister is domineering takes it to be true that the Prime Minister is domineering. The proposition taken to be true gives the content of the belief, which is simply what the subject believes. Someone who wants the Prime Minister to resign wants it to be true that the Prime Minister resigns. This time the propositional clause 'The Prime Minister resigns' specifies the content of a desire. The content of a belief is what would be the case if the

[1] See e.g. McGinn (1982*b*), ch. 1.

belief were true. The content of a desire is what would be the case if the desire were fulfilled.[2]

There is another distinction which cuts across that between sensations and propositional attitudes. A mental state may or may not be *conscious*, that is to say, being in that state may or may not be a feature of the subject's current consciousness. Sensations are always conscious in the sense of being episodes in the current stream of consciousness, though the subject may not always be conscious *of* them in the sense of noticing them. We may forget a back pain because absorbed in some activity, but it should not be inferred from this that while forgotten about the pain was not a conscious state. Pains are always features of consciousness, a fact which is sometimes expressed by saying that to have a pain is to feel a pain. However, as with other sensations the degree to which we attend to a pain may vary. Unlike sensations, propositional attitudes are not always episodes in current consciousness. At any given time some of our propositional attitudes are conscious and some are not. As I touch my coffee-mug I form the conscious belief that the coffee in it is cold. A few moments ago my current belief that my son is at school, which I undoubtedly held then, was not conscious. Similarly, I now have a conscious desire to make good progress in writing this chapter. A few moments ago my desire to see a film this weekend was not conscious.

Clearly sensory experiences are akin to sensations in so far as they are always conscious occurrences. On the other hand there are considerations which make it seem natural to classify them also as propositional attitudes. For instance, sensory experiences can be described in ways which involve the ascription to them of propositional contents. We can say that it visually seems to someone that *p*, meaning by that to describe how the person's experience represents the world as being without implying that the person believes or is even inclined to believe that *p*.[3] Also, it might be thought to be a fact about most

[2] This way of thinking about beliefs, desires, and kindred states is well set out in Dennett (1969), ch. 2. For a recent discussion with some distinctive twists, see Searle (1983).

[3] This manner of speaking can be found in e.g. McGinn (1982*b*), Searle (1983), and Peacocke (1979, 1983).

experiences that they would not be the experiences they are were it not that they essentially involve propositional contents. It is commonly said that when we see things we see them under certain descriptions. Looking at a rose-bush, for instance, you might see it as a rose-bush where this would imply that your visual experience would not be as it is but for its seeming to you that a rose-bush is there.[4]

Notwithstanding the considerations just mentioned, I shall argue in this chapter first, that if experiences are propositional attitudes then they must satisfy certain principles and secondly, that experiences do not satisfy these principles. The discussion will pave the way for an examination of epistemological topics.

Henceforth, when I speak of content I shall always mean propositional content and when I speak of experiences I shall always mean sensory experiences unless otherwise indicated.

1.2. *Experience, Perception, and Belief*

The notion of an experience needs some clarification at this point. Here and in what follows I shall for the most part focus on vision.

Suppose that you think you saw a black cat curled up in the corner of a room you have just passed through. Someone then leads you to doubt that there could have been a cat there. Despite this you may insist that, at any rate, when you looked in the corner of the room it was just as if there was a black cat curled up in the corner. Perhaps you did see a cat or perhaps it was just an illusion. Either way it was just as if you were looking at and thus perceiving a black cat curled up in the corner. This is a perfectly intelligible possibility and one which anyone with a grasp of the concept of perception can make sense of. I want to focus on the state which a person can be in when it is just as if he were looking at an *F* recognizing it to be an *F*. When you are in such a state you are having a visual experience *of an F*.[5] Some

[4] Related themes are explored in Hanson (1958).

[5] The idea that perceiving an *F* and having a perfect illusion of an *F* have something in common, variously described as an experience, sensation, or impression, or as one's being appeared to in a certain way, is shared by many writers who differ markedly in the accounts they give of the common element. See e.g. Ayer (1956), Chisholm (1957), Armstrong (1963), McGinn (1982*b*), Searle

philosophers prefer to speak in this context of having experiences *as of* such-and-such.[6] This locution would do as well though I shall not use it. The important thing is to distinguish between experience and perception. One may have an experience of an *F* yet not perceive an *F*. There is no pressing need to distinguish between experience *of* and experience *as of*.

The notion of an experience of an *F*, as just explained, and the notion of its seeming to you that an *F* is there might be taken to amount to much the same thing. However, for reasons which will emerge in Chapter 4 I shall distinguish the two. In the meantime I shall take it that the claim that an experience is of an *F* implies that it is such that it seems to the subject that an *F* is there. Furthermore, I shall take it that experiences of an *F* have the content ascribed by the corresponding seems-that clause.

There are two familiar ways in which we describe what people perceive. We say, for example, that Jenny saw that the milk was boiling over. It is natural to take this statement to entail that Jenny knew that the milk was boiling over on account of having a visual experience of milk boiling over. Jenny, we may suppose, was looking at a pan of milk, knew it to be a pan of milk, and saw the milk bubble up and run over the side of the pan. We also say, for example, that Jenny saw the intruder. Jenny may have seen the person in question in the street outside her house not knowing that he had just entered the house. She saw the intruder but did not recognize him as someone who had entered her house. The content of her visual experience was not that someone who had entered her house was before her but, let us suppose among other things, that a man in a navy-blue tracksuit was before her. To count as having seen the intruder either

(1983), Peacocke (1983). A dissenting voice is that of J. M. Hinton (1973). Hinton sets out various conditions on experience reports and argues that no reports we actually make satisfy the conditions. He concludes that in practice we do not work with a conception of experience which answers to experience reports conceived in line with the specified conditions. I find myself more convinced that the notion of experience as a common element of perception and perfect illusion is unproblematic than I am of either Hinton's conditions on experience reports or his claim that we do not make such reports. Later in this chapter I shall present a typology of experience which seems to me to be intuitively plausible and to harmonize with our ordinary thinking about perception. If experiences are as mysterious as Hinton makes out it ought to be very puzzling that such a typology is available. It should also be puzzling that a certain sort of memory involves the replay of past experiences. On this see 4.2.

[6] See e.g. McGinn (1982*b*) and Peacocke (1979, 1983).

this latter content or some other content possessed by the experience must have been true. The experience may also have had a content which was false, for instance, that the man had grey hair, but what matters is that it should have had some content which was true and that that content need not have been that an intruder was there. In general we can say that if you visually perceive *X* then you must have a visual experience having a content which is true of *X*. Similarly, if you visually perceive an *F* then you must have a visual experience having a content which is true of the *F* which you visually perceive. The circularity of this last formulation will be overcome in a moment.

My primary aim in this chapter is not the theory of perception but rather the theory of the content of experiences. I think it will be helpful none the less to have a more precise idea of how experiences relate to perception. With this in mind I shall formulate a plausible, if unrefined, version of the *causal theory of perception* as it applies to perceiving *X* and perceiving an *F*. According to this theory if you perceive *X* before you then at least the following must be true:

(1) *X* is before you.
(2) You have an experience which is caused by *X*'s being before you.
(3) That experience has a content which is true of *X*.

Similarly, if you perceive an *F* before you then at least the following must be true:

(1*a*) There is an *F* before you.
(2*a*) You have an experience which is caused by there being an *F* before you.
(3*a*) That experience has a content which is true of the *F* by the presence of which the experience is caused.

(3*a*) overcomes the circularity mentioned earlier.

The relation between experience and perception is strikingly analogous to that between belief and knowledge. One can believe that *p* without knowing that *p* and so also one can have an experience of an *F* without perceiving an *F*. If one knows that *p* then it must be the case that *p* and, as already noted, if one perceives an *F* before one there must be an *F* before one. If one knows that *p* then one must believe that *p*. Somewhat similarly, if one perceives an *F* then one must have an experience which if not of an *F* must nevertheless have a content which is true of an *F*.[7]

The analogy can be pressed further with the help of a simple account of *veridicality*. An experience of *X*/an *F* is veridical if and only if *X*/an *F* is before you. We are familiar with the point that true belief is insufficient for knowledge. It seems fairly clear also that veridical experience is not sufficient for perception. This has an important bearing on a thesis which John Searle has developed.[8] Searle claims that the contents of visual experiences have a *causal ingredient*. Thus the content of Tom's experience of a cup can be more adequately specified in the following way.

> Tom has an experience that (there is a cup before him and that there is a cup before him is causing that experience).

Just as the content of a belief is what would have to be the case if it were true, so the content of a visual experience is what would have to be the case if it were veridical. If Searle is right then Tom's experience would not be veridical unless there were a cup before him and there being a cup before him were causing his experience. This looks extremely odd since on the face of it there is no more reason to build a causal ingredient into the contents of experiences than there is to build such an ingredient into the contents of beliefs. Suppose that a crude version of the causal theory of knowledge is true according to which *A* knows that *p* only if *A* believes that *p* and his believing that *p* is caused by its being the case that *p*. It does not follow from this that *A*'s belief is true only if it is caused by its being the case that *p*. All that is required for the belief to be true is that it be the case that *p*. Supposing now that the causal theory of perception is true. In that case *A* perceives an *F* before him only if he has an experience of, say, a *G* and that experience is caused by there being an *F* which is a *G* before him. Again, it does not follow, nor surely is it true, that *A*'s experience is veridical only if it is

[7] The phenomenon of 'blind sight' (Weiskranz *et al.* (1974)) might lead one to doubt that having experiences in some modality is necessary for perception. Here I am concerned with conditions on ordinary perception. 'Blind sight' perception deserves to be called perception only in so far as it approximates to the ordinary case.

[8] See Searle (1983), esp. ch. 2. The discussion of Searle which follows is a modified version of parts of Millar (1985*a*).

caused by there being an *F* which is a *G* before him. The causal theory of perception does not by itself provide a reason to build a causal ingredient into the content of experiences and the analogy between experience and belief speaks in favour of the simple account of veridicality mentioned above.

A plausible conjecture about what leads Searle to his contrary position is that he fails to distinguish between veridical experience and perception. In terms of our example he seems tacitly to assume that Tom's experience will not be veridical unless he perceives a cup before him. Indeed I am inclined to think that Searle actually equates having a veridical experience of an *F* with perceiving an *F*. Granted the causal theory of perception it follows that for Tom's experience to be veridical it must depend causally on there being a cup before him. But then, the argument goes, since the content of an experience is what would have to be the case if it were veridical, the content of Tom's experience must contain the causal ingredient that the experience depends causally on there being a cup before him. Of course, this is not to say that Tom's experience would not have the content it does unless it depended causally on there being a cup before him, only that such a causal relation would have to obtain if the experience were veridical.

The problem with this line of reasoning lies in the initial move, that is, with the tacit assumption that Tom's experience is veridical only if he perceives a cup before him. But there is no good reason to accept this assumption. It is not difficult to think of examples which show that veridical experience is not sufficient for perception. They are just the sort of examples which motivated the causal theory of perception. Here is one. Suppose that when Tom has his experience of a cup he is actually looking through a hatch in a wall at a mirror whose edges he cannot see. Tom is unaware of the presence of the mirror and takes himself to be perceiving a cup located just where his experience suggests that a cup is. For the mirror is so angled that it reflects light from a scene involving a cup of the appropriate sort against the appropriate background. Suppose now that behind the mirror there is another scene involving a cup. This entire scene, if it were viewed from Tom's position, with no intervening mirror, would be in appearance the mirror image of the first scene if the latter were to be viewed straight on (that is from a position on a line of incidence from the scene to the mirror) and not via the mirror. The arrangement results in Tom's having an experience which is qualitatively identical to that which he would have were he to perceive the scene behind the mirror. Of course he does not perceive that scene for the requisite causal relation does not obtain. None the less it visually seems to Tom that there is a cup before him of a certain type against a certain background, and there is. So by the simple account of veridicality his experience is veridical.

Some people initially find it odd to think of Tom's experience as being veridical in the circumstances envisaged. The sense of oddness, I think, derives from two sources. The first is simply the fact that Tom's experience does not depend causally on the scene behind the mirror. But while that is a reason for saying that Tom does not perceive the scene behind the mirror, it is not a reason for denying that his experience is veridical in the sense explained. The second source of the sense of oddness is the fact that Tom's experience is deceptive. This is a more serious point. Its resolution reveals an important feature of the concept of veridicality. Tom's experience is of a cup of a certain type against a certain background. But it is also an experience of there being nothing (but air) between Tom and a cup before him. Since there is something, a mirror, before him the experience is deceptive and, surely, not veridical. This is correct. What it shows is that, as one would expect, veridicality is relative to specified content. *Qua* experience of a cup before him, Tom's experience is veridical. *Qua* experience of there being nothing between Tom and a cup before him, it is not. Tom's experience is deceptive but this does not undermine the simple notion of veridicality nor count in favour of Searle's.

There is a further line of thought in Searle's work which could be pressed into service at this point, although Searle does not rely on it when he introduces the view that the contents of experiences contain a causal ingredient.[9] Searle thinks that we are 'directly aware of causation in perception'. What he means is that whenever we have a visual experience, whether veridical or not, we experience it 'as caused by something independent of us'. In support of this Searle asks us to consider the following thought experiment.

[9] Searle (1983), pp. 123 ff.

Suppose we had the capacity to form visual images as vivid as our present visual experiences. Now imagine the difference between forming such an image of the front of one's house as a voluntary action, and actually seeing the front of the house. In each case the purely visual content is equally vivid, so what would account for the difference? The voluntarily formed images we would experience as caused by us, the visual experience of the house we would experience as caused by something independent of us. The difference in the two cases is a difference in the causal content of the two experiences.[10]

There is clearly something right about this. When we have a visual experience we instinctively believe it to be caused by something in our environment which we take ourselves to perceive. Such beliefs may be confirmed or disconfirmed by the ways in which the experiences in question cohere, or fail to cohere, with past and subsequent experience, both visual and in other modalities, in the way we should expect if the experiences were caused by what we think they are caused by. Visual images produced at will would not cohere, and would not be expected to cohere, in the right kind of way. So it seems plausible that there would be a difference in 'feel' between such images and the typical visual experiences of ordinary perception. The question though is whether this difference provides a reason to suppose that the contents of visual experiences contain a causal ingredient. On this I remain unconvinced. It seems more natural to regard the content of visual experiences or images as being exhausted by what Searle calls their visual content, the way things seem visually to the subject. Searle allows that voluntarily produced images and familiar visual experiences could have the same visual content, and he is right in thinking that the difference which he describes is not explained at that level. I think it can be explained in terms of differences in the memories and expectations which would be associated respectively with voluntarily produced images and the usual visual experiences. There seems to be no compelling reason to suppose that these differences require to be explained in terms of a difference in content of the sort envisaged.

In the next section I shall take up some further issues which are germane to Searle's views. The discussion thus far has emphasized that veridical experience is not sufficient for

[10] Searle (1983), p. 124 n.

perception and drawn attention to the importance of the notion that veridicality is relative to specified content. This last point, it should be noted, is a consequence of the fact that specifications of the contents of experiences are partial. In saying that an experience is of a cup we do not specify the kind of cup nor the kind of background or foreground. One and the same token experience may be of many things. It may be of an *F* and of a *G* (where the concept of an *F* and the concept of a *G* are different). A token experience of a cup might be at the same time an experience of a spoon. Thus while an experience of a complex state of affairs is a complex experience, it is not to be conceived as a complex of experiences.[11] We can therefore avoid consideration of how Tom's present experience of a cup combines with his present experience of a spoon. Such combination is not to the point. If Tom is looking at a cup and spoon his token experience of a cup is identical with his token experience of a spoon.

I shall now take a closer look at the idea that experiences, and in particular the sorts of experiences which figure in perception of the world, are propositional attitudes.

1.3. *Experience and Content*[12]

As indicated in the last section I assume that having an experience of an *F* is, at least in part, a matter of having an experience such that it seems to you that an *F* is there. It is time now to be a little more precise about what this latter notion amounts to. As I shall understand it an experience is such that *it seems to you that an F is there* if and only if you would believe that an *F* is there in the absence of countervailing considerations.[13]

[11] I owe this way of stating the point to Sellars (1968), pp. 26 ff. Sellars has a concept of an impression according to which a complex impression is a complex of impressions.

[12] The discussion of this, the following four sections, and some of the previous section, draw upon and substantially modify material in Millar (1985*b*). I am grateful to Mark Sainsbury for critical comments on that paper which led to some of the modifications. Throughout this and the next three chapters I also make use of Millar (1989).

[13] This formulation is close to that of Peacocke (1983). Peacocke speaks of judgement rather than belief but this implies conscious thought, which may not always occur when one takes one's experience at face value.

Countervailing considerations include anything which casts doubt on the reliability of the relevant sense-modality, or which suggests that the intervening medium is not suitable for accurate perception, or which, independently of these considerations, casts doubt on whether an *F* is present. If, as in the usual case, you do believe that an *F* is there this belief need not be a conscious thinking-to-yourself that an *F* is there.

There is no doubt that contents can be ascribed to the sorts of experiences we typically have in perception. This is precisely what happens when we describe an experience as being *of* something. But to settle the matter of whether experiences of a certain sort are propositional attitudes we need to look more closely into the conditions which must be satisfied by a state if it is to be a propositional attitude. To this end I shall introduce two principles, the *Concept principle* and the *Intrinsicality principle*. It is plausible to suppose that a state which is worthy of being called a propositional attitude must satisfy both of these principles.

The Concept principle states that if a concept is an ingredient of the content of a mental state then the subject of the state must grasp the concept. If, for example, you believe that your pet cat is a Russian blue then you must grasp the concept of a Russian blue. This seems intuitively plausible. What could it be to ascribe content to a belief if the subject of that belief lacks the conceptual prerequisites for grasping that content? But the proposal is not without difficulty. We do sometimes say that a person believes that *p* without implying that he or she has full mastery of all the concepts which are ingredients of the proposition that *p*. Many of us could be said to believe that Geiger counters are for measuring radiation though we lack full mastery of the concepts of a Geiger counter and of radiation. Young children may be said to believe that tigers are fierce before they realize that tigers belong to the cat family. So it might seem that the Concept principle requires modification.

I think that this view of the matter over-reacts to the examples cited. What the examples show is that belief reports of the form '*A* believes that *p*' sometimes overdetermine the content of the belief in question. To the extent that they do they inaccurately report what the subject believes. It is not that people sometimes fail to grasp what they may accurately be said to believe but rather that they do not believe what they are inaccurately reported as believing. Belief reports which are thus inaccurate may for all that be acceptable in ordinary parlance where it can be made clear in the context that the subject should not be imputed with a full grasp of the content clause of the report. Our appreciation of the need to qualify belief reports of this type shows that we are tacitly guided by the Concept principle.

The Intrinsicality principle states that if token mental states in a given category (belief, desire, or whatever) have different contents then they are of different state-types within that category. Thus if Kate's belief B is the belief that p and Fred's belief B' is the belief that q, and the proposition that p is not the same as the proposition that q, then B and B' are different beliefs in the sense of being of different belief-types. This merely regiments the common-sense thought that people have the same belief only if what they believe is the same.[14] States which

[14] This common-sense thought may seem to be problematic in view of a cluster of issues about content which have been prominent in recent literature. Suppose that (i) beliefs are the same if and only if they have the same content and (ii) contents are the same if and only if they have the same truth-conditions. Now the following is possible: At each of two distinct times t and t' a person could have a belief whose content would be expressed by his then saying 'The shop round the corner is open'. Yet it could be that the content thus expressible at t is true while that expressible at t' is false. In the interval between t and t' the shop might have closed. On the standard view of truth-conditions, contents which have different truth-values have different truth-conditions. So by (ii) the content of the belief at t differs from the content of the belief at t' and by (i) the beliefs must differ in that they are different beliefs. This is puzzling. It may be that nothing that we would ordinarily count as a psychological change in the subject has occurred between t and t' yet we seem forced to attribute distinct beliefs at t and t'. The issue is not one which can be resolved in a footnote. All I want to point out is that it does not demand revision of the Intrinsicality principle so far as beliefs are concerned. It has to be conceded that on the conception of content captured by (ii) the contents of the beliefs in the example differ. But there is a corresponding sense in which the beliefs differ. Nor is this altogether at odds with common sense. (Utterances of sentences like 'The shop round the corner is open' make tacit indexical reference to the time of utterance. They say in effect 'The shop round the corner now is now open.' Suppose utterances of 'p' and 'q' are of that sort and that neither 'p' nor 'q' contains explicit temporal indexical terms like 'now'. I think we have a fairly common-sense notion of difference of belief in accordance with which to believe at t that p is to have a different belief from that which one would have were one to believe at t' that q, where t and t' are distinct, if believing at t' that q would not commit one to believing at t' that at t p. This latter condition is obviously met in our example.) There is also a sense in which the contents in our example are the same, but then there is a corresponding sense in which the beliefs are the same, the sense which sustains the thought that no psychological change in the subject

satisfy the Intrinsicality principle may be said to have intrinsic contents in that possession of a particular content by a token state in a given category is intrinsic or essential to its being the type of state that it is within the category.[15]

If experiences are propositional attitudes then they must satisfy our two principles. Initially there seems to be no difficulty in the idea that experiences satisfy the Concept principle. Certainly it is true that if you have an experience of an *F* then you must possess the concept of an *F*. The general idea is clearly enunciated by Christopher Peacocke in the following passage.

> [I]t is in the nature of representational content that it cannot be built up from concepts unless the subject of the experience himself has those concepts: the representational content is the way the experience presents the world as being, and it can hardly present the world as being that way if the subject is incapable of appreciating what that way is.[16]

The matter is not quite as straightforward as this makes it seem. Part of what is at issue is whether being *of an F* can be an intrinsic feature of experiences.

Some comment is needed concerning the implications of applying the Intrinsicality principle to experiences. The basic idea is simple enough. Experiences which differ in content are different experiences, in the sense of being of different experience types. But what is it for experiences to be of the same or different types? One suggestion would be to answer this with

need have taken place between *t* and *t'*. So again the Intrinsicality principle is not impugned. There would be a problem if the only legitimate notion of belief content were that captured by (ii) and the only legitimate notion of sameness of belief were that which reflects the aforementioned intuition about psychological change. But I see no reason for thinking that true. Of course, detailed discussions of belief should make clear which notion of content is at issue when the principle is invoked. On related problems of content, see Putnam (1975a). For a useful analysis and an amusing example—The Ballad of Shakey's Pizza Parlour—see Dennett (1982). McGinn (1982*a*) contains a clear and useful perspective on the background theory. For an approach to the puzzle which I find congenial, see Fodor (1986).

[15] Note that if possession of the content that *p* is intrinsic to an experience's being of the type it is then it is also an intrinsic feature of the experience in the sense that in any possible world in which the experience occurs it has the content that *p*.

[16] Peacocke (1983), p. 7.

the help of what I shall call the *principle of phenomenal character*. This states that experiences are of the same (different) types if and only if they have the same (different) phenomenal character(s). Unfortunately, the suggestion does not take us very far since our grip on sameness and difference of phenomenal character is only as good as our grip on qualitative sameness and difference of experience. To answer our question illuminatingly we should need some independent account of phenomenal character. None the less the proposed principle is of some importance if it is read as supplying a constraint on adequate accounts of phenomenal character. I suggest that read in this way the principle is acceptable. It is difficult to see how the notion of phenomenal character could be illuminated except in terms of some prior grasp of what it is for experiences to be alike or different *qua* experiences.

It is of some interest to note that Searle violates the principle of phenomenal character. He wants to allow for the possibility that two experiences have the same phenomenal character and yet one is of Sally and the other is of Sally's identical twin sister.[17] This latter difference is a difference in content and so, Searle thinks, differences in content may not be reflected in differences in phenomenal character. But he also appears to accept the Intrinsicality principle and to hold that visual experiences satisfy it. As he puts it, 'the two forms of mental phenomena, belief and visual experience, are intrinsically Intentional. Internal to each phenomenon is an Intentional content that determines its conditions of satisfaction'.[18]

Let us assume, at least for the sake of argument, that visual experiences can have contents which their subjects could express by saying 'Sally is before me' or 'Sally's twin is before me'. Searle's view has it that although, by the Intrinsicality principle, an experience of Sally and an experience of Sally's twin would be different they might none the less be the same in phenomenal character, which violates the principle of phenomenal character. Since Searle does not accept that principle he would not see this as an objection to his view. But the question remains whether Searle has given us a good enough reason to

[17] See Searle (1983), p. 50.
[18] Ibid., p. 40.

reject a principle which has powerful intuitive appeal, and to this the correct answer, in my view, is negative.

Consider what it might be like to have successive experiences on looking at Sally and then at her visually indistinguishable twin. Assume that the point of view is the same, that both women are dressed in exactly the same way and in exactly the same pose against exactly the same background. Now there clearly is some sense in which you may see Sally as Sally and Sally's twin as Sally's twin. You may have appropriate background beliefs as a result of which on having the one experience you are led to believe that Sally is there and on having the other experience you are led to believe that her twin is there. I find it odd to suppose that such a difference amounts to a difference in the intrinsic features of the experience, a difference in the experiences *qua* experiences. Searle's view of the matter is that you could have an experience of Sally the content of which has a causal ingredient to the effect that the experience is caused by the presence of Sally and a phenomenally identical experience of Sally's twin the content of which has a causal ingredient to the effect that the experience is caused by the presence of Sally's twin.[19] Thus although such experiences would be phenomenally identical they would have different intrinsic features because they differ in content. But this line of thought turns on the thesis that the contents of visual experiences have a causal ingredient, which, as I argued in the last section, is not well motivated. There are in any case other responses to the example which Searle does not consider. One might deny that experiences can have singular contents. The consequence would be that while an experience can be *of a woman* it could not be *of Sally*.[20] Alternatively, one might hold, as against Searle, that there is after all a phenomenal difference between the two experiences.[21] Both of these responses would be consistent with

[19] See Searle (1983), pp. 62 ff.

[20] See McGinn (1982*b*), pp. 38 ff.

[21] This is the line taken in Peacocke (1983). Searle may seem to be committed to it by his view, discussed in the previous section, that we are directly aware of causation in perception. If he is then the commitment does not fit comfortably with his explicit treatment of the experiences of Sally and of her twin. But it is not clear that he does incur the commitment in question. To experience causation when we have a visual experience may just be to have a sense of the experience's being caused by something independent of one, rather than the sense of its being caused by this or that in particular. If this is how we are to

retaining the principle of phenomenal character and the view that experiences satisfy the Intrinsicality principle. But there is yet another strategy: reject the view that experiences must satisfy the Intrinsicality principle and retain the principle of phenomenal character.

This is the line which I shall defend in the following sections. I shall do so with the help of examples which do not involve singular contents. The thesis to be argued implies that token experiences may differ in content yet not be different *qua* experiences (phenomenally, qualitatively). The thesis allows for the possibility that token experience *E* is such that it seems to its subject that an *F* is there and yet is of the same type as a token experience *E*' which is not such that it seems to its (possibly different) subject that an *F* is there. Obviously it is incumbent on anyone who takes this view to spell out the relevant typology. We must ask again what it is for experiences to be of the same or different types. This is what led to the discussion of the principle of phenomenal character, but as yet no adequate answer has been forthcoming.

1.4. *A Typology of Experience*

A good starting-point is to consider pains rather than sensory experiences. Everyone knows that there are distinctive kinds of pain. The pain produced when you touch a flame is different from the pain produced in your elbow after a blow to your funny-bone, which in turn is different from the pain produced when you have a cramp in your toes. Most people will have had these types of pain and will know which type is referred to by the descriptions of the circumstances in which they are produced. Some specifications of types of pain mention an event which would usually result in the pain being felt. Others mention some accompanying circumstance such as the peculiar dislocation of toes in which one has cramps. Yet others mention

understand the matter then there need not be phenomenal differences between experiences corresponding to differences in their causal ingredients. By the same token it is puzzling that Searle should think that experiences have specific causal ingredients at all.

some peculiar behavioural symptom such as wincing after having drunk something cold which affects a bad tooth.

Let us regiment specifications of the type of a pain of the sort illustrated as follows:

A's pain is of the type produced when/if . . . .

where the gap is filled with a description of producing causes, accompanying circumstances, peculiar symptoms, or whatever.[22] Someone might now suggest that while such specifications are all very well in that they, so to speak, indicate the type of a pain, they do not say what type the pain is. The thought underlying this suggestion is that knowing that a pain is of the type produced when/if such-and-such occurs is not yet to know *which type* it is. A more philosophical version of essentially the same thought would be that specifications conforming to our regimented form merely indicate the type of a pain but do not describe its phenomenal character. But at this point we have to ask what a proper description of a pain, one which brought out its phenomenal character, would be like. Certainly, we describe pains as dull, sharp, throbbing, or blinding, and as having varying degrees of intensity, but such descriptions lack the specificity and range of application of type specifications along the lines of our regimented form. In describing pains there is no getting round descriptions of the publicly observable circumstances in which they are produced.

One way of responding to this last point would be to claim that we know what pains are like simply by having them. The idea here is that through introspection we can have knowledge of the phenomenal character of pains, knowledge which is not articulable in the form of descriptions. So although there is no better method of indicating the type of a pain than those currently being discussed it remains true that these methods fail to describe the phenomenal character of pains as known by their subjects. I agree with those who have thought that this line of thought rests on a fundamental error; that of regarding the mere having of an experience of a certain type as knowledge of the

[22] The basic idea here is familiar in functionalist accounts of mental states. See e.g. Churchland (1984). The idea, developed below, of specifying types of sensory experiences via circumstances which would normally produce them is used in Sellars (1956, 1968). See also Churchland (1979).

phenomenal character of experiences of that type.[23] It is this error which is at the root of the thought that our regimented specifications do not say what type a pain is.

Yet there is an important connection between knowing what it is like to have a pain of a certain type and having pains of that type. If you have never had the distinctive type of pain produced when your funny-bone is struck then you will not know what it is like to have a pain of that type. This point, however, has no tendency to show that descriptions of our regimented form do not capture the phenomenal character of pains. It would do so only if you could grasp what is said by someone who tells you that the pain in their elbow is the type produced when one's funny-bone is struck, but not know what type of pain that is. But if you do not know the type referred to you would not grasp what you are told. No more would you grasp the statement that some man is the type who wears polo necks and drives a Volvo, if you do not know which type that is.

The next step is to extend the essential idea behind the pain typology to sensory experiences. This seems quite natural. We can describe a visual experience as being of the type you get when you look at a car or, more specifically, at a blue car from the left-hand side on a sunny day. We can describe a tactile experience as being of the type you get when you run your hand over a sheepskin rug. We can describe a gustatory experience as being of the type you get when you taste something with garlic and rosemary in it. In each of these cases it would be just as odd as in the pain case for someone who has had experiences of the type in question and who has associated experiences of that type with the circumstances described to ask, 'And which type is that?' Such a person will know what phenomenal character the experience described has in virtue of knowing it to be of the type you get when/if . . . .

At this stage it will be useful to have available a rather more formal presentation of the suggested typology so far as it applies to sensory experiences. In what follows I shall assume, as hitherto, that '*F*' is a schematic letter which stands in place of general substantival terms which convey the typical appearance, to

23 See Sellars (1956) and, more recently, Rorty (1980), ch. 4 sect. 3. I take it that the error in question is one which Wittgenstein was concerned to expose in Wittgenstein (1958).

the relevant sense-modality, of the things to which they apply.

Let us say that an experience in the modality of *M* (sight, touch, etc.) is *F-type* if and only if it satisfies the following condition: in suitable environmental conditions an *F* would produce an experience of that type in an observer who is suitably positioned and orientated and whose sense of *M* is normal. As rough shorthand I shall say that *F*-type experiences are ones which *F*s (would) *yield* or, alternatively, ones which you (would) get if *F*s (were) are accessible to the modality in question. Thus a visual experience might be (red thing)-type or, more interestingly, (apple on a tree)-type. A tactile experience might be (rough and hairy thing)-type. An aural experience might be (clap of thunder)-type.

Some clarificatory remarks are in order. First, the condition for being *F*-type contains a modal element; it refers to conditions which would produce an experience of the type in question. This means that we can meaningfully describe an experience using a concept which is empty so long as the use of the concept conveys the appearance of the sorts of things which, if they existed, would be its instances. Thus we might properly describe a visual experience as being dragon-type. Secondly, although *F*-type experiences are ones which *F*s yield it does not follow that usually when one has an experience of that type it is produced by an *F*. In other words, *F*-type experiences are not necessarily, as I shall say, *F-indicating*. In a world in which there are realistic plastic potted plants (potted plant)-type visual experiences might as often as not be produced by things which are not potted plants but only look like them. Thirdly, numerically distinct token experiences which are both *F*-type may differ *qua* experiences (phenomenally, qualitatively) in many ways. One may be (*F* which is *G*)-type and the other not, or one may be (*F* against background *B*)-type and the other not. Note that an experience which is (*F* . . .)-type, where the gap is filled in with some further specification, is also simply, though not, of course, merely, *F*-type.

The proposed typology admits of an interesting refinement. The descriptions which take the place of '*F*' may be regarded as straightforward descriptions of environmental situations. But there are some types of experience which cannot be adequately characterized unless mention is made of some particular condition of the subject. An example would be the sorts of experiences you can have when you make yourself see double. Suppose you look at a cup while making yourself see double. The experience you have is one which a cup would yield to an observer who is making himself see double. I shall say it is (cup [as seen double])-type. Another example would be (cup [as seen with eyes screwed up])-type. Yet another, in a different modality, would be (voices [as heard with ears full of water])-type. A particularly interesting class of cases, which I discuss further in I.7, concerns looking at things with an artist's eye with a view to discerning, for instance, the shape aspects which they present. Thus looking at a cup rim in this way you might notice that it presents an elliptical aspect. Here, I would say that the experience you obtain is (cup [as seen with a view to discerning shape aspects])-type. In general, an experience in the modality of *M* is (*F* [as perceived . . .])-type if and only if it satisfies the following condition: in suitable environmental conditions an *F* would produce an experience of that type in an observer who is suitably positioned and orientated, whose sense of *M* is normal, and who via *M* is perceiving an *F* . . . . Here the gap is to be filled by a specification of a special condition of the subject of the sort illustrated.

This last definition makes it important to read the normality condition on the relevant sense-modality in a way which is broad enough to allow that, for example, one's sense of sight is normal even when one is looking at something with screwed up eyes. This reading is also important in that it enables us to think of experiences which are (*F* [as perceived . . .])-type as special cases of experiences which are *F*-type.

A problem to which this sort of typology gives rise is that of giving a non-circular account of what suitable environmental conditions and suitable positioning and orientation are. Suitability, one is tempted to say, is suitability for producing *F*-type experiences, but we were trying to say what *F*-type experiences are. What I have in mind is that suitability is suitability for perception, though not necessarily recognition, of things of the type in question. This as it stands would make any account of perception of an *F* in terms of *F*-type experiences circular, but this is a circularity we can put up with. A scientific account of perception would be expected to yield an account of what the relevant conditions are which makes no mention of perception. By making it clear that suitability is suitability for perception I intend to indicate that, for example, in the case of cup-type experiences the range will include the sort of experience you might have if you were to glimpse a cup out of the corner of your eye as well as the sort you might obtain if you were to look straight at a cup. In the case of a (grouse in grass)-type experience the intended range would exclude experiences obtained when looking straight at a grouse which is completely camouflaged by its colouring and background. We have general ideas of the sorts of conditions of the environment and of subjects which permit perception, if not necessarily recognition, in various sorts of case. It is these ideas which give some bite to the notions of suitable environmental conditions and of suitable position and orientation of the subject.[24]

I have already suggested that the typology of sensory experience, which I shall call the *F*-type typology, is similar to the proposed typology of pains. The latter is very clearly implicit in our ordinary talk of pains. If the *F*-type typology seems to be less familiar this is due in large measure to the fact that in our ordinary thinking we perhaps do not talk very much about what our experiences are like. None the less I contend that it comes naturally to us when we think about our experiences. Apart from that, a grasp of the typology is implicit in our ordinary talk of the appearances of things relative to the various modalities. That is to say it is implicit in our ordinary talk of the look, or sound, or feel, or smell, or taste of things.

If you know what a thrush looks like (the look of thrush, how a thrush looks) then, I contend, you must have an idea of the sorts of experiences you have when thrushes are in sight. This means both that you must have had thrush-type experiences and have an idea of such experiences as being the ones which thrushes yield. The argument in support of this view is as follows. It is uncontentious that you cannot know the look of a thrush unless you have enjoyed thrush-type experiences. But to

[24] Some types of experiences are not accommodated by the scheme thus far. For instance, certain types of migraine result in a blind spot in the visual field. The experiences obtained in this condition are apt for perception but one's sense of sight could hardly be said to be normal while the condition obtains.

know what something looks like you must not only have come by the appropriate experiences, you must have the notion of them as being the appropriate experiences. The reason is that knowing what an *F* looks like is a matter of being able to recognize *F*s and things with similar visually perceptible characteristics, and that means being able to judge of things perceived whether they are or are not visually *F*-like. Being in a position to make such judgements on the basis of visual experiences in turn requires a grasp of when such judgements can be justifiably made and when not, and that requires a grasp of the sorts of experiences which put one in the position to make the judgements. It is not an implication of this view that experience-based judgements are justifiably made only when the subject has considered the experiences in question. The point is rather that knowing when one is in a position to make judgements in a certain class involves essentially an ability to appraise judgements in the class, whether made by oneself or others, with respect to whether or not they are justified, and in the case of experience-based judgements that ability requires one to know the sorts of experiences the having of which would in the absence of countervailing considerations warrant such judgements. So there is no knowing what thrushes look like, and thus being able to make visual experience-based judgements to the effect that a thrush or something visually thrush-like is there, without a notion of the sorts of experiences which are thrush-type.

I shall be looking much more closely at the epistemology of experience-based judgements in Chapter 4 where further light will be shed on the preceding line of thought. I shall in the meantime assume that the argument is sound and that we have a grasp of the *F*-type typology of experience in so far as we have a grasp of similarities and differences in the look of things. This last point holds good even for the refined version of the typology which takes account of peculiar conditions in observers in the manner explained earlier in this section. Just as we can talk of the look of thing *simpliciter* so we can speak of the look of a thing when observed in a special way or when the observer satisfies some particular condition. Thus at all points our thinking about looks harmonizes with the proposed typology.

1.5. *Experiences, Concepts, and Recognition*

There is nothing in the notion of an *F*-type experience which requires subjects of such experiences to possess the concept of an *F*. In this respect sensory experiences are analogous to pains. You can have a pain of the type produced by cramp in your toes even if you lack a concept of pains of that type. By contrast, you cannot have an experience such that it seems to you that an *F* is there unless you have the concept of an *F*. Recall that an experience is such that it seems to you that an *F* is there when it is such that in the absence of countervailing considerations you would believe that an *F* is there. To be in such a state clearly you must have the concept of an *F*. It follows that an *F*-type experience may not be such that it seems that an *F* is there.

To illustrate the point imagine that Charlie Brown has the concept of a pumpkin. He can distinguish pumpkins from other fruit in the supermarket. He knows that they are fruit and come from certain kinds of bush. His friend Jimmy, who lives in a remote corner of Scotland, has no concept of a pumpkin at all. He has no idea of what they look or taste like and doesn't even know that they are fruit. Suppose now that Charlie and Jimmy were in turn to look at a pumpkin from the same point of view in conditions suitable for perceiving pumpkins. In all likelihood Charlie would have an experience which is both pumpkin-type and such that it seems to him that a pumpkin is before him, for this is what he would believe in the absence of countervailing considerations. But since Jimmy lacks the concept of a pumpkin it cannot seem to him that a pumpkin is before him. Nevertheless, Jimmy could have a pumpkin-type experience.

The distinction between an *F*-type experience and an experience such that it seems that an *F* is there enables us to express succinctly the manner in which experiences interact with conceptual capacities. Roughly speaking, the idea is that for a person who has a mastery of the concept of an *F*, *F*-type experiences are apt to be experiences such that it seems to the subject that an *F* is there, where that is explained by the capacities constitutive of mastery. To have a mastery of the concept is to possess capacities such that given *F*-type experiences as input one is disposed to believe that an *F* is there in the absence of countervailing considerations. To be thus disposed by an experience is for it to seem to one that an *F* is there. We can also be more precise about what it is for an experience to be *of an F*. An experience is of an *F* when it is both *F*-type and such that it seems to the subject that an *F* is there.[25]

At this point we need to take account of an important refinement concerning concepts. Thus far the only restriction I have placed on substituends for '*F*' is that they should convey the typical appearance to the relevant modality of the things to which they apply. Now a term may convey the typical appearance of things of a certain class even if it is not possible to tell that something is a member of the class from its appearance. Thus the term 'apple' conveys the typical visual appearance of apples, but if there were as many visually apple-like non-apples as apples it would not be possible to tell that something is an apple from its visual appearance and apple-type experiences would not be apple-indicating. In that case for those who knew this to be so apple-type experiences would not be apt to be experiences such that it seems that an apple, as opposed to something which merely looks like an apple, is there. Now if the concept of an *F* is to be a suitable ingredient of the content of experiences in some modality it seems reasonable to suppose that the corresponding conceptual capacity must be suitable for interaction with *F*-type experiences in the way suggested above. That is to say, the capacities constitutive of mastery of the concept of an *F* must be such that for a subject who has these capacities *F*-type experiences are apt to be experiences such that it seems that an *F* is there. For that to be true the concept of an *F* must satisfy the condition that its mastery enables one to tell that something is an instance from its visual appearance. It will emerge in Chapter 4 that further refinements are necessary.

With these various preliminaries in mind let us return to the crucial question raised towards the end of 1.3, the question whether experiences satisfy the Intrinsicality principle. I shall defend the view that they do not. The issue should now be much clearer than it was. If experiences do satisfy the Intrinsicality principle then the following Special Intrinsicality principle holds: If distinct token experiences have different contents then

[25] In Ch. 4 I consider cases in which experiences which are not *F*-type are nevertheless experiences such that it seems to the subject that an *F* is there.

they are of different types. With the *F*-type typology to hand we are better able to appreciate what this means, but we need to proceed with care. I remarked in the last section that distinct token experiences which are both *F*-type may differ in that, for instance, one is (*F* which is *G*)-type and the other not. Any plausible typology of experience would have to accommodate a parallel claim. This being so it cannot be assumed that two token experiences are of the same type, in the sense of being phenomenally identical, simply in virtue of both being, say, *F*-type. I take it that experiences are of the same type, in the sense of being phenomenally identical, if and only if there is no type such that one is of that type and the other not. I shall also take it that two experiences may be said to be of different types if and only if there is some type such that one experience is of that type and the other not. If there is some type such that distinct experiences are of that type then I shall say that the experiences share a type.

We saw that in the Charlie Brown example Charlie and Jimmy could have experiences which share a type, in that both are pumpkin-type, though only Charlie's experience could be such that it seems to him that a pumpkin is there. But, assuming that the concept of a pumpkin is suitable as an ingredient of the contents of visual experiences, the defender of the Special Intrinsicality principle is committed to a much stronger claim, namely that if Charlie's and Jimmy's experiences differ in content, in consequence of the different conceptual equipment of Charlie and Jimmy, then these experiences cannot be of the same type. The claim here is that since the contents differ the experiences must differ *qua* experiences.

What are the differences supposed to be? I hope that by now it is clear that it will not do simply to point out that Charlie's and Jimmy's experiences will differ in that Charlie will perceive the pumpkin as a pumpkin while Jimmy will not. My view allows that there is a sense in which this is so which turns on the fact that Charlie's experience is of a pumpkin while Jimmy's is not. What the defender of the Special Intrinsicality principle must show is that this difference must reflect a difference in phenomenal type. There is no doubt that we can make sense of the thought that there need be no difference. The thought is simply that while both Charlie and Jimmy have experiences of the same type in the sense explained, only Charlie's experience is such that it seems to him that a pumpkin is there. This latter feature of Charlie's experience is to be conceived as being extrinsic to its phenomenal character. For the experience to have the feature is a matter of its disposing Charlie to believe that a pumpkin is before him in the absence of countervailing considerations. So it is perfectly intelligible to suppose that while Jimmy's experience is just like Charlie's it does not dispose him to believe that a pumpkin is there because it does not interact with the required conceptual equipment.

The defender of the Special Intrinsicality principle need have no difficulty in acknowledging that Charlie and Jimmy could each have pumpkin-type experiences. But he will suggest that none the less the experiences must differ. In effect he thinks of the difference as being due to what in the previous section I referred to as special conditions of the subject. In this case the special conditions are conceptual capacities of the subject which are supposed to affect the phenomenal character of experience. But whereas we have a good idea of how our visual experiences are affected by screwing up our eyes or making ourselves see double, it is less easy to say how they are supposed to be affected by exercising a conceptual capacity. At this point the defender of the Special Intrinsicality principle is likely to appeal to certain familiar facts about experience and recognition. You may suddenly recognize the face of someone who has been in sight for some time. It is not just that you come to be in a position to judge that the person is so-and-so. You see the person in a different way, in a sense which implies that there has been a phenomenal change in your visual experience. Similarly, it would be argued, the experience of a person who on looking at a pumpkin recognizes it to be a pumpkin would be different from that of a person who looks at the pumpkin in exactly the same conditions but does not recognize it as a pumpkin.

The point can readily be granted, but more is needed to vindicate the Special Intrinsicality principle. Let us vary the example. Suppose that for some time you have had in view a black cushion-like object in the corner of a sofa. Suddenly, you realize that it is a cat curled up with its head well tucked in. As you recognize the cat as a cat your visual experience changes phenomenally. The defender of the Special Intrinsicality principle must hold that the experience you have after you recognize the cat as a cat could not be the way it is unless you had recognized the cat as a cat. His aim is to show that the content that a cat is there is intrinsic to the type of the post-recognition experience. But that goes further than the facts of the matter require and has difficulties of its own. The facts are consistent with the suggestion that the phenomenal change in experience has to do with a change in the salience of certain features of the cat. As your eyes play over the cat, focusing on different parts of it, the ears, the texture of the fur, and so forth, become salient. It seems quite plausible that this change in salience, far from being dependent on your recognizing the cat as a cat, actually explains how you came to recognize the cat for what it is. The contrary view, that the phenomenal change is essentially dependent on recognition, makes it seem mysterious that recognition should have taken place at all.

By way of reply it might be argued that the notion of salience smuggles in recognitional capacities. Perhaps you recognize the cat because you recognize the features mentioned. So even if you do not need to possess the concept of a cat in order to have the kind of experience in virtue of which you were able to recognize the cat as a cat, nevertheless, the argument would go, unless you had concepts of the relevant features you could have no such experience. The problem with this reply is twofold. First, it simply is not clear why salience has to be conceived in terms of full-blooded recognition, that is, recognition understood in the familiar way as involving the application of concepts. Salience in the visual case is a matter of the extent to which an object or feature stands out against a background. Thus a grouse which is camouflaged by grass would not be salient, but a pumpkin in full view alone on a shelf very likely would be. There is no reason to suppose that salience in this sense demands full-blooded recognition. Perhaps the liability of an object or feature to be salient for you may be dependent on your past experience and in particular on your exposure to the object or feature in question. But it would be a further and dubious step to argue that past experience can only affect current experience via the exercise of conceptual capacities.[26]

[26] Learning can affect one's experience by refining one's capacity to attend in detail to things perceived. See Goldstein (1984), pp. 188 ff. Those who have

The second problem for the proposed reply is that it does not address the problem of how recognition can take place. On any view of the matter recognition arises from the interaction of incoming experiences and standing conceptual capacities. There has to be something about the experiences which explains their being apt to trigger recognition and that cannot be something which is essentially dependent on recognition having taken place.

The relation between experience and recognition has featured prominently in discussions of ambiguous figures. Famous examples include the drawings of the duck/rabbit, the vase/faces, and the old woman/young woman. Similar effects are produced by numerous types of fragmentary figure, usually collections of black blotches which come to be seen as a drawing of something familiar. It is characteristic of such examples that as one looks at the drawing one sees it first in one way and then in another. Moreover, the changes in ways of seeing are genuinely visual. It is not just that you come to realize that what you see admits of a certain description.[27] Malcolm Budd speaks of such cases as involving seeing something in accordance with first one interpretation then another. He suggests that 'the intrinsic nature of seeing something in accordance with an interpretation does not have an essence that is capable of being specified independently of the interpretation'.[28] I take it that this is to be understood as implying that the character of the experience is not independent of the content of the interpretation. The experience would not be what it is without the content of the interpretation. If this were right then our experience of these figures would create a difficulty for the view I have developed.

There is a more and a less radical response to this. The less radical response is simply to concede the point but note that it fails to show that in general the contents of experiences are intrinsic to the types of these experiences and thus does not sustain the view that experiences in general are propositional attitudes. The more radical response, which I favour, calls into

learned to focus their attention on the taste of wines have a capacity to recognize types of wine which others lack. But the fact that learning can affect the way people attend to wine which in turn affects the concepts they can apply to wines does not show that the contents of their experiences of wines are intrinsic.

[27] For useful descriptive material and analysis, see Rock (1983).

[28] Budd (1987), p. 13.

question whether the content of the interpretation in accordance with which a figure is seen really is intrinsic to the type of the experience involved.

What seems to require that certain contents are intrinsic to the successive experiences obtained when looking at, say, the duck/rabbit drawing? There seem to be two principal considerations. One is that we cannot specify the difference between the two experiences except in terms of the two different descriptions in accordance with which the figure is seen. This will not do the trick for it leaves open the possibility that although we need to use the descriptions 'drawing of a duck' and 'drawing of a rabbit' to characterize the experiences, we need not use them as content specifications in the sense understood in this chapter. Why should we not think of the successive experiences as being, in whatever order, (drawing of a duck)-type and (drawing of a rabbit)-type, yet without having as intrinsic contents, respectively, the proposition that a drawing of a duck is there and the proposition that a drawing of a rabbit is there? This is where the other consideration comes in. It is thought to be especially puzzling to suppose that we can conceive of the possibility that the successive experiences could be divorced from the contents in question because recognition seems to be essentially involved. It is supposed not to be clear what it would be to have the experience one has when one sees the figure as a drawing of a duck unless, in something like my sense, it seemed to one that a drawing of a duck were before one.

On the other hand things are not plain sailing for the view that the experiences in question have intrinsic contents. If the content that a drawing of a duck is there is intrinsic to the experience had when one sees the figure as a drawing of a duck then having such an experience essentially involves the exercise of mastery of the concept of a drawing of a duck. But it is not clear that or why mastery of the concept of a drawing of a duck need be thus involved. Wouldn't the concept of a duck do or just the concept of something having those characteristics which, as it happens, make a thing visually duck-like?[29]

[29] Tom Bower, in Bower (1985), ch. 7, reports studies which show that children who have never come across pictures can apply the names of familiar objects to their pictorial representations. He argues that this does not show that the children in question must have a notion of the representations as representations of the familiar objects.

What does seem to happen in these cases is that the figure we are looking at takes on a form with which we are familiar. The question is whether we are compelled to account for our sense of familiarity in terms of full-blooded recognition. Obviously, if in looking at the duck/rabbit figure one acquires a belief that it is like a drawing of a duck or like a duck then the corresponding conceptual capacities must be engaged. But as in the cases previously considered we still need to explain what prompts recognition when it does take place. In the cat-on-the-sofa case I suggested that certain features of the cat become salient and it is this which accounts for recognition. I want to suggest now that something similar occurs in the cases under consideration. A certain form stands out and this enables those of us with the appropriate conceptual capacities to see the figure as having the form of a duck or the form of a rabbit. But we can make some sense of the idea that such a form may stand out even for one who lacks appropriate conceptual capacities. Imagine a young child who prior to having much understanding of language, and certainly prior to having learned to use the names 'duck' and 'rabbit', shows fear in the presence of ducks but not in the presence of rabbits. If on being presented with a life-size drawing of the duck/rabbit figure the child shows fear we would have some, if not conclusive, grounds for thinking that the child had something like a duck-type experience.[30] One could imagine other sorts of reaction which would further support that conclusion. The experience in question would be identified via its functional role—it is produced by vaguely duck-like things including, sometimes, duck/rabbit drawings, and it produces certain reactions and behavioural dispositions.

Clearly in our thought experiment the duck-form has a certain significance for the child—it prompts fear. But a disposition to experience fear on having a certain type of sensory experience hardly amounts to a conceptual capacity. In later chapters I favour the view that to possess a concept is to have a pattern-governed capacity to form, maintain, and evaluate beliefs whose contents include the concept. The capacity is pattern-governed in that its exercise is guided by certain patterns, including inference patterns. My hunch is that the phenomenal switches

30 Psychologists studying children often make inferences to the sort of experience a child is having from behavioural reactions. See Bower (1985), ch. 3.

associated with our experiences on looking at ambiguous figures involve capacities which are much more basic than conceptual capacities in the sense explained.[31]

It might be suggested that my doubts about the Special Intrinsicality principle rest on an unduly restrictive phenomenology of experience. An adequate phenomenology, it might be said, would recognize that when you have a visual experience of an *F* your preparedness to believe that an *F* is there, in the absence of countervailing considerations, suffuses your experience and contributes to its being the experience it is. To my mind there are at least two difficulties with this. One is simply that it seems to give your preparedness to believe a role in your current stream of consciousness which it may not have. How is it supposed to figure in consciousness if not in the form of a thought to the effect that what is before you is an *F*, or would be if the experience were veridical? Yet such thoughts need not be present when having an experience of an *F*. The other difficulty is that even if it were conceded that the preparedness in question does figure in your stream of consciousness that would not settle the matter of whether it was essential to the type of the visual experience. For all that has been argued it would remain possible that a component in the current stream, namely the visual experience, is of a type which may be shared by tokens which do not occur in conjunction with the preparedness to believe that an *F* is there.

John McDowell has attacked the view that intrinsic features of experiences are vehicles of extrinsic representational contents. This position, he says, 'would have it that the fact that an experience represents things as being one way rather than another is strictly additional to the experience's intrinsic nature, and so extrinsic to the experience itself'.[32] McDowell adds that if

[31] Psychologists working with information-processing models of the mind commonly distinguish between top-down processing and bottom-up processing. Top-down processing is usually taken as being cognitively or conceptually driven while bottom-up processing is data driven. See e.g. Goldstein (1984), ch. 7, and Bruce and Green (1985), ch. 4. I have been raising doubts about whether top-down processing needs to be posited to account for *Gestalt* switches. To this extent I follow the general spirit of Fodor (1983). However, nothing I have said implies that the character of sensory experiences is fixed purely by output delivered at an early stage in the visual system. Past experience may affect current experience via mechanisms quite high up the visual system which none the less fall short of being conceptual or cognitive.

[32] McDowell (1985), p. 116.

this view is correct then it would seem natural to speak of representational contents as being 'read into' the experiences of which they are contents. His objection to the view is that it falsifies the phenomenology and cannot explain how contents can be read in. This line of thought is instructive in that it reveals one source of the difficulty which some philosophers find with the idea that the phenomenal character of an experience can be divorced from its content. I take it that the worry is essentially twofold. First, if content has to be read into an experience this would imply that the subject in some way consciously considers the experience. But no such consideration need take place when people perceive things. Secondly, it is left obscure how the subject is supposed to interpret the experience so that it can be understood as representing some objective state of affairs.

McDowell seems to me to be quite right in thinking that the metaphor of 'reading in content' leads to insuperable difficulties but the view that contents are extrinsic to experiences does not license its use. To say that the content that *p* is extrinsic to the type of a token experience is simply to allow for the possibility that a distinct token may be of the same type yet not bear the content that *p*. This does not entail that those for whom the experience does bear the content that *p* must in some way have read it in. The picture is rather that in virtue of having the right concepts such people are disposed on having experiences of the relevant type to believe that *p*, in the absence of countervailing considerations.

Kant famously said that intuitions without concepts are blind.[33] Some philosophers might be tempted to suppose that experiences without concepts would be, well, very different from the experiences we actually have in that they would be 'unorganized' mosaics of colour and shape and would lack depth features.[34] It may forestall possible misunderstanding to stress that the typology I have proposed concerns the fully

[33] See Kant's *Critique of Pure Reason* B75 in the Kemp-Smith trans., Kant (1933), p. 93.

[34] O'Shaughnessy (1980), i. 171 ff., argues that visual sensations 'form a 2D array in psychological space', using as an assumption the thesis that 'concepts play a causal role in the genesis of visual depth experience'. In support of the assumption he says that 'any visual depth experience depends upon seeing one's visual sensations as contributing the colour of physical items situated at some distance from one'. O'Shaughnessy's visual sensations are not the same as my visual experiences. They are meant to be the 'given' element in perception.

'organized' experiences with which we are all familiar. There is on my view a real sense in which experiences without concepts would be blind. It is only through the exercise of capacities one has in virtue of possessing concepts that experiences can represent the world as being one way rather than another and can contribute to the justification of beliefs. Experiences without concepts might enable a creature to react differentially to its environment, but would not on that account give the creature a perspective on its environment which it could itself evaluate and correct. Such a view is consistent with the negation of the Special Intrinsicality principle.

1.6. *Admissible Contents*

In this section I shall consider an objection to the view I have developed. It might be suggested that the problem in the Charlie Brown example is created not by the application of the Intrinsicality principle to visual experiences but rather by too loose a view of the sorts of contents which experiences can have. Speaking of sensory experiences Colin McGinn has said that we should 'restrict the concepts invoked to characterise content to those that relate to the appearances of things—concepts of colour, superficial texture, shape etc.'.[35] The restriction is meant to be understood in such a way that it rules out the concept of an *F* as a possible ingredient of the contents of experiences in the modality of *M* if it is possible that there are things which, though not *F*s, have the appearance of *F*s relative to *M*. The rationale is supplied by the desideratum that the contents of experiences should deal with properties which are 'fully manifest to the senses'.[36] That something is a tiger is not fully manifest to sight, for instance, since there is more to being a tiger than having a certain visual appearance, so there is a sense in which to specify the content of an experience as being of a tiger overdetermines any possible phenomenal character it

The trouble is that in so far as they figure at some level prior to the formation of fully blown experience it seems inappropriate to describe them as sensations and inappropriate to talk of seeing sensations as . . . .

[35] McGinn (1982*b*), p. 40.
[36] Ibid.

might have. A description of an experience as being of a tiger requires it to be no different phenomenally from an experience described merely as being of something having the look of a tiger.

The same would apply to other natural-kind concepts like that of a pumpkin. The objection now under consideration is that given a view of admissible content along the lines suggested by McGinn the Special Intrinsicality principle can be sustained. The argument might be along the following lines. Precisely because a description of an experience as being of a pumpkin over-determines its phenomenal character an experience obtained looking at a pumpkin need not represent to the subject that a pumpkin is there. The idea here is that it makes no difference to the intrinsic character of the experience whether it is of a pumpkin rather than merely of something having such-and-such visible properties. When Charlie looks at the pumpkin he has an experience of something having such-and-such visible characteristics. Jimmy is not precluded from having such an experience for want of the concept of a pumpkin. Suppose then that the conceptual ingredients of experiential contents are restricted as on McGinn's account. The suggestion then is that whereas we can make sense of the idea that a normal visual experience such as would be obtained on looking at a pumpkin by someone who has a concept of the visual appearance in question might not be of a pumpkin, we cannot make sense of the idea that an experience of the same phenomenal character might not be of something having the visual appearance in question. Stated thus baldly the argument assumes the point at issue, but it is open to a more satisfying criticism.

When concepts are applied in perception the subject incurs commitments to how the thing seemingly perceived would look from points of view other than those which he currently occupies. To illustrate this consider the concept of something having the visual characteristics which happen to be those of a pumpkin. I shall call this the concept of a visually pumpkin-like thing, or alternatively, the concept of something having the look of a pumpkin. As I shall use these locutions in this section, a person may possess the concept in question though not possessing the concept of a pumpkin. They are convenient abbreviations in place of locutions which spell out the colour, shape, size, and visible texture of a pumpkin. The concept does meet McGinn's standard of admissible content for there is no question of a thing's having the appearance of being visually pumpkin-like but not being visually pumpkin-like. But what matters for our present purposes is the application of the concept in perception. On the view that I favour a person who applies the concept in perception incurs commitments to how the thing to which it is applied would look from diverse points of view. Indeed, to apply the concept in perception is just to believe that something in view would look various ways from various points of view. Clearly it is possible for the concept to be competently applied to something which is not an instance because it would not look the way instances should when further inspected. So beliefs to the effect that an instance is present, formed while perceiving something from a particular point of view, are subject to correction in the light of experiences obtained through further inspection. Now it is conceivable that a person should look at something visually pumpkin-like from a certain point of view yet lack any conception of what the thing would look like from other points of view. A person who lacked the concept of a visually pumpkin-like thing would be in just such a situation. According to the Special Intrinsicality principle, the experience obtained by such a person on looking at a pumpkin could not be phenomenally the same as that obtained in the same way by a person who was exercising the relevant conceptual capacity. But it is difficult to find a rationale for this view given the present account of concept application. If to apply the concept in perception is just to believe that something in view will look such-and-such ways from various points of view then there seems no reason to suppose that the experiences which an instance yields should be affected by whether or not the subject possesses the concept. In other words, the nature of the relevant conceptual capacity does not explain why applying the concept in perception from some point of view need affect the experience obtained from that point of view.

The obvious, if rather tiresome, next step would be to fall back on the concept of something having a side like that of a pumpkin, where that is taken to be a concept of the visible properties of the side of a pumpkin. But essentially the same problem remains. A thing might look like something having a side like that of a pumpkin, but not be something having a side like that of a pumpkin, because it does not continue to look that way from distances of more than, say, ten feet. And we can conceive of someone faced with something having a side like that of a pumpkin not having the usual expectations about what it would look like from distances greater than ten feet. The problem is to say why the lack of such expectations should affect the current visual experience of such a subject.

The problem I have identified is a general one. For any concept applicable to perceived objects or scenes it will always be possible that something which is not an instance presents to a given point of view an appearance which is just like that which an instance would present to that point of view. Correspondingly, it always seems intelligible that a person presented with an appearance from one point of view should lack the usual expectations about what an instance of the concept should look like from other points of view. The problem is to see why lacking these expectations should affect the way the object looks from the given point of view. And if that is a problem then there is a problem over how it makes a difference to the way the object looks from the given point of view whether the subject exercises the conceptual capacity in question.

The same point holds for straightforward colour concepts. When you have an experience of something red you are disposed in the absence of countervailing considerations to apply the concept of a red thing, not to some two-dimensional shape hovering in your visual field, but to something out there in the environment before you capable of presenting the appearance of being red to certain points of view without being red. Certainly, if a thing has the appearance, the look, of being red, in the intended all-round sense, then it is red. For in the intended sense a thing does not count as having the look of something red unless it yields appropriate courses of experience on inspection in suitable conditions. But a thing can have the look of being red to a certain point of view and not be red. So again we seem to be able to conceive of someone faced with something red yet lacking the usual expectations about what it would look like from other points of view. And the problem again is to see why that should make a difference to the phenomenal character of the experience.

I shall say a little bit more about colour concepts in order to counter possible objections. The view which I have been developing in the last few sections allows that a (red thing)-type experience can fall short of being an experience of a red thing. Some people may still feel unease about this on the grounds that if a person were capable of displaying those reactions which would warrant attributing to him a (red thing)-type experience, then it would follow that he would have, and would be exercising, mastery of the concept of a red thing. This would create a difficulty for the idea that a (red thing)-type experience could fall short of being an experience of a red thing.

The objection can be met with the help of an example. Suppose that Fred has been brought up in an unusual environment and in a rather extraordinary way. In his environment there is only one red thing, a wooden block. Fred has never learned to use colour words, but people sometimes point to the block asking him to fetch it, which he does. Perhaps it is called by a proper name with which Fred is familiar. When people refer to the block using this name and ask Fred to fetch it, he does. How does Fred know that the block is referred to in either of these ways? Well, we may suppose that it is salient against the backgrounds in which it is usually kept and that it has been picked up and handled and talked about by others in Fred's presence. It would be clear to Fred that he has fetched the thing intended if those who have asked him to fetch it seem satisfied when he does. While all of this shows that Fred can discriminate the block, in the sense of visually picking it out from its backgrounds, it does not show that Fred must be able to recognize the block as something red. For one thing recognition of the block as something red involves the ability to distinguish between something's merely appearing to be red in certain conditions of illumination and its actually being red. Nothing we have ascribed to Fred guarantees that he has an appreciation of that distinction. But despite this there is every reason to think of him as subject to (red thing)-type experiences. These are just the sort that people obtain when they look at red things and Fred shows all the signs of having them in so far as he can locate the block relying on sight.[37] Of course, Fred cannot think of

[37] Tony Pitson, in Pitson (1984), writes that '[t]he condition that what is seen should be discriminated or differentiated from its environment points to a

himself as a subject of (red thing)-type experiences, but that does not mean that he cannot enjoy such experiences.

The example serves as a further illustration of a point made in the last section. A feature can be salient to a subject who has no concept of that feature as such and thus no ability to form and evaluate beliefs concerning it. A subject can register the presence of a feature *Q* through having an experience with a feature which correlates with the presence of *Q* and which is apt to have an impact on the subject's behaviour. But having such an experience may fall short of its seeming to the subject that something having the feature *Q* is present. I conclude that colour concepts present no special difficulty for the line which I have been pursuing.

That completes the main line of argument of this chapter. I have articulated and defended a conception of sensory experiences according to which these experiences do not satisfy the Intrinsicality principle and thus should not be conceived as propositional attitudes. In Chapter 4 I shall take up the question of how sensory experiences thus conceived contribute to the justification of beliefs. In the concluding section of this chapter I briefly discuss a further matter concerning the character of sensory experiences.

1.7. *Sensational Properties*

Peacocke has argued that experiences have sensational properties as well as representational contents. As noted earlier (1.3) he thinks that experiences satisfy the Intrinsicality principle. However his views about sensational properties are independent of that principle and of interest on their own account. I shall develop and modify them to some extent and briefly consider how the possession of sensational features by an experience relates to its type as conceived in the *F*-type typology.

cognitive element in seeing' (pp. 128–9). I do not deny that there is a cognitive element in seeing if by that is meant that perception essentially involves being in states which have intrinsic propositional contents. This much is accommodated by the rough account sketched in 1.2. The point in the text is simply that there is a sense in which we can discriminate or pick something out by its colour even if we have no concept of the appropriate colour properties.

Peacocke gives the following example:

> Suppose you are standing on a road which stretches from you in a straight line to the horizon. There are two trees at the roadside, one a hundred yards from you, the other two hundred. Your experience represents these objects as being of the same physical height and other dimensions; that is, taking your experience at face value you would judge that the trees are roughly the same physical size. . . . Yet there is also some sense in which the nearer tree occupies more of your visual field than the more distant tree. This is as much a feature of your experience itself as its representing the trees as being the same height. The experience can possess this feature without your having any concept of the feature or of the visual field: you simply enjoy an experience which has the feature.[38]

The feature indicated by saying that the nearer tree occupies more of the visual field than the more distant one is what Peacocke calls a sensational property. Of course, trees do not, strictly speaking, occupy visual fields. An experience could possess the feature in question even if there were no scene present of the kind described. Peacocke provides the outline of a convenient and economical way of expressing such features, which I shall develop slightly. Let us say that a region *R* of the visual field of a token experience *E* is the *phenomenal counterpart* of a region *S* of physical space provided that if the circumstances were normal what appears in the region *R* of *E* would be explained principally by what occupies *S*.[39] We can now introduce the relation of *being larger' than* as follows. Imagine a plane perpendicular to the subject's line of vision. A region *R1* of the visual field is larger' than a region *R2* of the visual field if *R1* stands to *R2* in that relation which in normal circumstances would be produced by two objects *X* and *Y* satisfying this condition: *R1* is the phenomenal counterpart of the space occupied by *X* and *R2* is the phenomenal counterpart of the space occupied by *Y* and the area of the interposed plane which would have to be opaque to obscure *X* is larger than the area which would have to be opaque to obscure *Y*. By this account the area of the visual field occupied by the nearer tree is larger' than the area occupied by the farther tree.

[38] Peacocke (1983), p. 12.

[39] The notion of a phenomenal counterpart is used more broadly in Sellars (1968).

Peacocke rightly stresses that this fact is not captured by specifications of the content of the experience. The experience (as I would say) is of a row of trees of equal height stretching away from one in a straight line, and much else besides, none of which brings out the distinctive sensational property described. One might have an idea of what it is to have an experience of such a scene yet fail to realize that such experiences have the sensational property in question.

Other sensational properties may be introduced in an analogous way. For example, a region *R* of the visual field is *elliptical'* if it has that property which in normal circumstances would be produced by an object *X*, say, the rim of a cup, which occupies the space of which *R* is the phenomenal counterpart, and which would be precisely obscured by an elliptical region of the imagined interposed plane. Sensational colour properties can be introduced too. A region *R* of the visual field is *red'* if it has that property which in normal circumstances would be produced by a red object occupying the space of which *R* is the phenomenal counterpart.

This method of introducing sensational colour properties has its shortcomings. It masks the fact that there are sensational properties which relate to redness in much the same way as the property of being elliptical' relates to being circular. The rim of the cup is circular and looks circular. The experience you would usually have if you were to look at it would be of a circular cup rim. Nevertheless the rim would present an elliptical aspect to most points of view. Were you to capture this aspect in a drawing you would do so by means of an ellipse. This is not to say that the rim looks elliptical. On the contrary, it looks circular and would continue to look circular through changes in the aspects it presents. (This is the phenomenon of shape constancy.) Presenting an elliptical aspect is a property which the rim could be perceived to have by any normal observer looking at it from my point of view and attending to the shape aspect which it presents. Attention is required because we do not as a matter of course notice the shape aspects which things present even when we perceive the things themselves and perceive that they have the particular shapes that they do. That is one reason why it is difficult to draw. The experience you have when you look at a cup rim in the ordinary way from a point of view to which it presents an elliptical aspect is actually different from that which you would obtain if you were to attend to the aspect from the same point of view. Nevertheless there is a sense in which the experience you have when you look at the cup rim in the ordinary way could be said to register an elliptical aspect. This is just another way of stating that there is an elliptical' region in the visual field. Analogous points hold for colours. The plastic penholder on my desk is a uniform shade of red but presents a vast range of colour aspects through changes in my point of view and through changes in the prevailing conditions of light. Each such aspect is a richly textured pattern of light and shade. Throughout changes of aspect the penholder continues to look a uniform shade of red. (This is the phenomenon of colour constancy.) Looking at it in the ordinary way one might not notice the aspect it presents. Yet the experience I have as I look at it from some point of view under particular conditions of light registers the colour aspect which it presents to that point of view in these conditions. The experience is not on that account *of that aspect* any more than the ordinary sort of experience of the cup rim is *of an elliptical aspect*. The method of primed predicates does not enable us to handle properties such as these with precision. We do not have a fine-grained vocabulary for describing colour aspects themselves and so have no systematic way of introducing sensational properties corresponding to particular colour aspects.

The discussion of colour and shape aspects reinforces the point made earlier to the effect that sensational properties are not captured either by content specifications or by type specifications. A stronger point also holds. The subject of an experience would not in the ordinary course of events know which sensational properties his experiences have. Such knowledge requires mastery of the relatively sophisticated concepts which are expressed by primed predicates. A subject of an experience which possesses a sensational property is not bound to possess a concept of that property. This may seem to give rise to a difficulty. It may be thought puzzling that an experience can have a feature which contributes to its being the kind of experience it is, if the subject does not know that the experience has the feature. This line of thought is seductive but it overlooks the crucial distinction between features of consciousness and what one is conscious of. When I look at the red penholder I am conscious of a red penholder simply in virtue of having an experience of a red penholder. But my experience also registers the particular aspect of red that the penholder presents. Registering this aspect is a sensational property of the experience and as such is certainly a feature of my current stream of consciousness. The experience would not be what it is if it registered some other aspect of red. It would be a mistake, however, to assume that if the property in question is had by an experience then it must be one of which the subject is conscious. On the contrary, while such properties can be said to affect the manner in which we are conscious of things they need not be properties of which we are conscious.[40]

Peacocke thinks that there are cases of *Gestalt* switch in which the sensational properties of succeeding experiences are held constant and their representational content changes.[41] He gives as an example the three-dimensional wire cube. One experience presents the *ABCD* face of the cube to be in front of the *EFGH* face, while the other presents the reverse to be the case. The experiences register the same shape aspects in the same region of the visual field, yet there is undoubtedly a difference in the phenomenal character of the experiences. Peacocke's view is that at the level of sensational properties the experiences are the same. The difference in their phenomenal character is a difference in their representational content.

However, the example does not show that the noted difference in phenomenal character needs to be explained in terms of a difference in content. Although successive experiences register the same shape aspects in the same region of the visual field it by no means follows that they are the same in respect of all their sensational properties. And in fact there does seem to be a difference. To spell it out we need to introduce the sensational property of *being behind*'. A region *R1* of the visual field is behind' a region *R2* of the visual field if *R1* stands to *R2*

[40] Compare the following remark by D. W. Hamlyn: 'What might be said is that [sensations] give a kind of character to the form of awareness of the object even when one's attention is not directed to them . . . when it is the features of the object that grip our awareness and attention that awareness is still coloured, as it were, by the sensations that may so easily come before our attention.' From 'Unconscious Inference and Judgment in Perception' in Hamlyn (1983), pp. 26–7.

[41] See Peacocke (1983), pp. 16 ff. and 22 ff.

in that relation which would normally be produced by two objects *X* and *Y* satisfying this condition: *X* occupies the region of space of which *R1* is the phenomenal counterpart, *Y* occupies the region of space of which *R2* is the phenomenal counterpart, and *X* is behind *Y*. In the case in hand one experience is such that the region of the visual field which is the phenomenal counterpart of the space occupied by the *ABCD* face is behind' the region which is the phenomenal counterpart of the space occupied by the *EFGH* face. The other experience is such that the region of the visual field which is the phenomenal counterpart of the space occupied by the *EFGH* face is behind' the region which is the phenomenal counterpart of the space occupied by the *ABCD* face.

How then do sensational properties relate to experience types as I have conceived them? There are two crucial considerations here. One is that there are types and sensational properties such that necessarily an experience of that type has that sensational property. For example, an experience of the type which a circular cup rim at an oblique angle yields will necessarily register an elliptical aspect. The other consideration is that the same sensational property may be instantiated in experiences of very diverse types. An elliptical aspect may, for example, be registered by an experience which is (stylized drawing of a fish)-type. Let us say that an experience which is *F*-type belongs to the experiential type *T*(*F*). We can then formulate a relation between sensational properties and experiential types as follows. An experience type *T*(*F*) belongs to the type class of a sensational property *P* if and only if *F*-type experiences necessarily have *P*. This formulation allows that very diverse experience types may figure in the type class of a sensational property. Thus the property of registering an irregular parallelogram aspect has a type class which includes some experiences of the type *T*(thing having a rectangular surface) as well as experiences which are not of that type, for instance, some experiences belonging to the type *T* (thing having a surface with the shape of an irregular parallelogram). This is because experiences having the property in question can be produced by situations containing rectangular-shaped things as well as by situations lacking such things but containing instead things which have the shape of an irregular parallelogram.

2

Reasons, Justification, and Evidence I

2.1. *Reasons and Justification*

In the previous chapter I was concerned with topics in the philosophy of mind. In this and the next I turn to topics in the theory of knowledge. The two sets of topics will be brought together in Chapter 4 where I shall consider whether, and if so how, experiences contribute to the justification of beliefs.

The beliefs to be considered are believings of particular subjects rather than propositions which are or might be believed. It is clear that at least some beliefs are justified because of relations which they bear to other beliefs. They are, one might say, derivatively justified. Thus your belief that *p* may derive its justification from your beliefs that *q*, *r*, and so forth. The general epistemological framework which I shall adopt is best conveyed by considering a number of conditions on derivatively justified belief.

One plausible condition can be stated as follows:

JUS1 *A*'s belief that *p* derives its justification from his beliefs that *q*, *r*, . . . only if *A*'s belief that *p* is based on his belief that *q*, *r*, ...

This is what I shall call the *Basing condition*. Basing is to be understood as a causal notion.[1] If your belief that *p* is based on your belief that *q* and your belief that *r* then you believe that *p* because you believe that *q* and believe that *r*. For example, you may believe that a colleague is around the department because, looking over at his office-window, you believe that the light is on in his room and you also believe that whenever the light is on

[1] See Armstrong (1973), pp. 77 ff., Goldman (1979), and Swain (1981), ch. 3.

he is around. In this example, an experience-based belief, that the light in your colleague's room is on, and a standing belief that whenever your colleague's light is on he is around, bring it about that you believe your colleague to be around. It would be a mistake, however, to suppose that whenever a belief is based on others the subject came to have it because of these others. Basing has to do not just with the acquisition of beliefs but with their maintenance. It might be true of you now that you have a standing belief that your colleague is around because you now have other standing beliefs to the effect that he was around earlier and that whenever he was around earlier he continues to be for the rest of the working day. But you may not have acquired the belief that your colleague is around because of the beliefs on which it is now based. You may have acquired that belief in the first place on looking over at his room, but you now continue to believe that he is around, and your belief is sustained rather than brought about by the beliefs on which it is based.

To deal with basing which has to do with the maintenance of beliefs Armstrong makes use of a distinction between efficient causes and sustaining causes.[2] Efficient causes are events which bring about other events. Sustaining causes are states of affairs which maintain other states of affairs in existence. For example, the table's being underneath and in contact with the cup maintains the cup's staying where it is. As we have noted, sometimes when a belief is based on others it is not brought about by these others but is sustained by them. Armstrong observes that the relevant notion of sustenance is weak sustenance. A belief weakly sustains another if it is sufficient, though perhaps not necessary, to maintain it in existence. This copes with cases in which the causation of a belief is overdetermined. I shall assume that we need some such notions as these to characterize the basing relation.

Obviously, the Basing condition *JUS1* is not sufficient for derivative justification. We need also a *Rational Connection* condition. There has to be some sort of rational or reason-giving connection between the basis beliefs, that *q*, *r*, . . . , and the belief for which they are the basis, the belief that *p*. Let us experiment with the following:

[2] See Armstrong (1973), pp. 79 ff.

JUS2 *A*'s belief that *p* derives its justification from his beliefs that *q*, *r*, . . . only if the proposition that *q*, the proposition that *r*, . . . constitute a reason for thinking that *p*.

Ignoring scruples about the use of symbols, I shall abbreviate the right side of *JUS2* by saying that *q*, *r*, . . . constitute a reason for *p*. It is worth taking some time to elucidate the concept of a reason-for-thinking since it will loom large in what follows.

The relation in question is to be taken as holding between propositions or, more precisely, between a series of propositions and some further proposition. Roughly speaking, *q*, *r*, . . . is a reason for *p* if *p* may be inferred from *q*, *r*, ...[3] Although the premisses of a deductively valid argument do constitute a reason for its conclusion, not all legitimate inferences are deductively valid. At any rate, if our Rational Connection condition is to be at all plausible and if the notion of a reason is to be linked as suggested with that of inference, then there are going to have to be inferences the legitimacy of which is not a matter of their being deductively valid. We shall be looking at examples shortly.

Our ordinary talk of reasons reflects a wide range of concepts. The abstract notion of a reason-for-thinking, which is the primary concern here, must, for instance, be distinguished from that of a *reason why* a person believes something. Reasons-why are causes and the cause of a belief will usually be other beliefs or some combination of beliefs and experiences. We also speak of a person as having a *reason to believe* something. You have a reason to believe that *p* if *q*, *r*, . . . is in the abstract sense a reason for *p* and you legitimately take it for granted that *q* and that *r*, and . . . . Having a reason to believe in this sense is sometimes expressed in terms of having grounds for belief. Note that you may have a reason (grounds) to believe that *p* even if you do not believe that *p*.

A reason to believe that *p*, in the sense just explained, is always a good reason. Often we speak of *a person's reasons (or grounds) for believing* something in a sense which allows for the possibility that the reasons (or grounds) may be bad as well as the possibility that they may be good. In this sense your reasons

[3] There are weaker notions of reasons. See e.g. Blackburn (1973), ch. 2.

for believing that *p* comprise the contents of the beliefs which form the basis of your belief that *p*. Basing the belief that *p* in this way may not satisfy either the Rational Connection condition or the Basis condition which I shall consider shortly.

Among reasons in the abstract sense it is important to distinguish between *unconditional* and *conditional* reasons. *q, r,* . . . constitute an unconditional reason for *p* if *p* may be inferred from *q, r,* . . . *without further ado,* that is to say, without relying on further assumptions as premisses along with *q, r,* . . . . The premisses of a deductively valid argument constitute an unconditional reason for its conclusion. Our ordinary ways of speaking show that we have some grasp of another kind of reason, a conditional reason. It is quite natural to speak of inferring that a copper bar will expand from the fact that it is being heated. Although the inference cannot be made without further ado, it is taken as read that all copper expands on heating and this proposition, together with the assumption that the bar in question is being heated, constitutes an unconditional reason for thinking it will expand. Conditional reasons are context-relative in that they hold only in contexts in which appropriate further premisses may legitimately be taken for granted. With this in mind we may say that *q, r,* . . . constitute a conditional reason for *p* relative to a context *C* provided that there are further propositions which may be legitimately taken for granted in *C* and which, together with *q, r,* . . . , constitute an unconditional reason for *p*.

The distinction between conditional and unconditional reasons enables us to strengthen *JUS2*. It is to be understood that the basis beliefs from which a belief that *p* derives its justification are adequate for the justification of the belief that *p*. That is to say, they are causally sufficient to bring about or maintain the belief that *p*, and their contents are in a sense rationally sufficient. The thought here is that the belief that *p* does not merely derive its justification in part from the beliefs that *q, r,* . . . . We can capture this thought with the help of the following amendment to *JUS2*.

JUS2' *A*'s belief that *p* derives its justification from his beliefs that *q, r,* . . . only if *q, r,* . . . constitute an unconditional reason for *p*.

Suppose that *q*, *r*, . . . constitute only a conditional reason for *p*. In that case *A* would have to be able legitimately to take for granted some proposition or set of propositions which together with *q*, *r*, . . . constitute an unconditional reason for *p*. But then *A*'s beliefs that *q*, *r*, . . . would not be an adequate justificational basis for the belief that *p* and so, in the intended sense, that belief would not derive its justification from the beliefs that *q*, *r*, ...

JUS1 and *JUS2'* demand that a certain abstract reason-for-thinking relation holds between the content of the derivatively justified belief and the contents of the beliefs on which it is based. Their combined effect is to require that the causal link between the belief that *p* and the beliefs that *q*, *r*, . . . should mirror an appropriate series of inferential steps leading from the premisses *q*, *r*, . . . to the conclusion *p*. None the less, for all that has been said this mirroring could be a fluke. There is nothing to require that the inferential links between the propositions has anything whatsoever to do with *A*'s believing that *p* because he believes that *q*, *r*, ... But if it is a fluke then it would seem that *A*'s belief that *p* would not derive justification from the beliefs on which it based. Let us call this *the problem of the accidental rational connection*. In the next section I shall consider how it might be solved.

2.2. *Inferential Competence*

Recall the example in which, believing that whenever your colleague's light is on he is around, and seeing that his light is on, you come to believe on that basis that he is around. Both the Basing and Rational Connection conditions are obviously satisfied. Consider now why you might form the belief that your colleague is around on the grounds that you do. It is quite likely that you would have a certain belief-forming habit: If you take it for granted that whenever *p*, *q*, and you have a sufficiently pressing interest in whether *q*, then if you see that *p*, you conclude that *q*, unless other beliefs prevent you from doing so. When I say that you conclude that *q* I do not mean that you have engaged in a series of reflections in which you satisfy yourself that you may conclude that *q* on the grounds specified. I conceive of the exercise of such habits as resulting in the unreflective formation of beliefs. In the example you simply see that the light is on and form the belief that your colleague is around. Even allowing for further refinements it seems plausible that you could have a habit which is closely akin to that described.

The point which needs to be stressed is that it would be no accident that you acquired the habit in question. You would have learned to form beliefs in that way as you acquired a mastery of the logical concept expressed by the 'whenever — — —, ***' construction, for it would seem to be partially constitutive of such mastery that the subject knows how to employ the concept in circumstances such as those in the example. In forming your belief that your colleague is around on the grounds you do, you are, we might say, exercising a certain inferential competence, since competence in the employment of the concept is plausibly conceived as involving a grasp of its inferential role.

The inferential role of a concept is characterized by certain patterns of legitimate inference. Thus the logical concept expressed by the 'whenever — — —, ***' construction is characterized in part by the pattern:

Whenever *p*, *q*.
p
―――――――――
q

It is of some importance to bear in mind that instances of this pattern are inferences in the abstract sense. That is to say, the instances comprise a series of propositions which count as premisses and a proposition which is a conclusion from these premisses. I shall often use the term 'inference' in this abstract sense rather than in the psychological sense which implies a transition from beliefs to beliefs.

There is a great deal more to inferential competence than emerges from the 'colleague' example. But already we have in prospect a solution to the problem of the accidental rational connection. Let us say that a set of legitimate inference patterns underwrites the fact that *q*, *r*, . . . constitute an unconditional reason for *p* if *p* may be inferred from *q, r,* . . . by a series of inferential steps each one of which instantiates a pattern in the set. Using this notion we can formulate the following *Competence* condition.

JUS3 · *A*'s belief that *p* derives its justification from his beliefs that *q, r,* . . . only if *A*'s believing that *p* on the basis of his beliefs that *q, r,* . . . is an exercise of competence on his part with respect to a set of patterns of inference which underwrites the fact that *q, r,* . . . constitute an unconditional reason for *p*.

I have already stressed that a plausible account of justified belief will have to countenance legitimate inferences which are not deductively valid. We shall come across inferences of this sort shortly. In the meantime we must take a closer look at the notion of competence. The idea I shall explore is that competence with respect to an inference pattern is a matter of being governed by that pattern. It is by no means a trivial task to work out what this amounts to.

Let us say that a set of propositions which can figure as premisses of an inference which instantiates a pattern *K* of legitimate inference constitutes an *input* to *K*. Any corresponding conclusion is an *output* of *K* given those premisses as input.[4] We might be tempted to suggest that to be governed by *K* is to be so disposed that by and large whenever you accept a series of propositions which constitutes an input to *K* you also accept corresponding outputs. But there are two obvious problems with this. For one thing there is no reason to think that we should have dispositions of this sort. Assuming we acknowledge the legitimacy of the pattern

$$\frac{p}{\text{Either } p \text{ or } q}$$

it would be absurd to suppose that we should or could believe the infinitely many disjunctions which are corresponding outputs for each input proposition which we believe. And in

[4] In some cases, e.g. conjunction elimination, there is more than one output for a given input.

any case, why should we actually accept a proposition just because it may be inferred from other propositions we accept by a single inferential step? As Harman has observed,[5] it seems positively desirable not to clutter our minds with trivialities. The other problem, also noted by Harman, is that even if we accept a proposition because we accept certain others it may be that other information we have makes it reasonable to reject the proposition in question. My description of the belief-forming habit which figured in the 'colleague' example was designed to accommodate these points. In the example it is assumed that you are *interested* in whether your colleague is around, and that none of your beliefs prevents you from accepting that he is. Perhaps then if you are governed by a pattern *K* then, if you accept a series of input propositions to *K* and you have a sufficiently pressing interest in whether some corresponding output proposition is true, then by and large you will accept the output proposition unless other beliefs prevent you from doing so.

There is no doubt that we may fail to accept a proposition which may be inferred from others we accept even when we have a strong interest in whether it is true. For instance, we may not appreciate that there is an appropriate inferential relation between the relevant propositions because a complex series of inferential steps is involved. The proposal under consideration, however, is concerned solely with one-step inferential links between input propositions and corresponding output propositions, instantiating patterns which it is psychologically realistic to suppose that we are governed by. Still, it seems quite possible that we may fail to appreciate the joint relevance of propositions we accept to an issue in which we have an interest, and it would be implausible to attribute that failure in all cases to some kind of incompetence. In the 'colleague' case the ease with which you conclude that your colleague is around is partly explained by the fact that you have a certain routine for checking that your colleague is around. This ensures that the joint relevance of the proposition that whenever your colleague's light is on he is around, and the proposition that your colleague's light is on, will be salient for you on the various occasions when you go

[5] On this and the next problem, see Harman (1984), p. 108, and (1986), ch. 2.

through the routine. To cope with the general problem we must add a qualification to the effect that the joint relevance of the input propositions must be salient. By this I do not mean that you must think to yourself that these propositions are jointly relevant. The idea is rather that you are, as it were, primed so that it is likely that your beliefs in these propositions become appropriately active so as to generate a belief in a relevant corresponding output proposition.

I have been concerned to describe a belief-forming habit, but clearly the sort of competence we are seeking to characterize must also have to do with the maintenance of beliefs and the abandonment of beliefs. We imagined that having come to believe that your colleague is around you might continue so to believe, not because you check from time to time that his light is still on, but because your belief is sustained by your believing that he was around earlier and that whenever he was around earlier he continues to be around for the rest of the working day. These causal links would be explained by your having the following habit: if you believe that *q* and have a sufficiently pressing interest in whether *q*, you do not stop believing that *q* in the absence of specific reasons to do so, provided that you continue to believe that *p* and that whenever *p*, *q*, and the joint relevance of these propositions continues to be salient.

Another case is where you abandon your belief that whenever your colleague's light is on he is around, when you discover on some occasion that although his light is on he is at home. The habit here might be something like this: you give up a belief that whenever *p*, *q*, if, while you have a sufficiently pressing interest in whether it is true, you come to believe both that *p* and that not-*q* and the joint relevance of these propositions is salient.

I shall assume that to be governed by a pattern of inference essentially involves having habits of forming, maintaining, and abandoning beliefs, or, in short, habits of *belief management*, along the lines described. But a crucial element is missing in the account thus far, if it is to be of use in explicating what is involved in mastering concepts. This is the idea that if you are governed by a pattern of inference *K* then you will appreciate the legitimacy of inferential links which instantiate *K*. We need not assume that you can formulate *K*, but you must have a certain recognitional capacity: faced with propositions constituting an input to *K* and a corresponding output proposition, you are capable of recognizing that the latter may be inferred from the former without further ado. That you have such a capacity would be evidenced by your performing well on the sort of test in which you have to indicate whether given inferences are legitimate or not. If you have the recognitional capacity associated with being governed by K you should give the right answer for instances of *K*.[6] Your having the capacity in question would also be evidenced by the fact that in ordinary uncontrived situations you count inputs to *K* as unconditional reasons for the corresponding outputs. Given this recognitional capacity you can take account of inferential links instantiating *K* in various ways. You might do so, for instance, in considering whether to accept propositions which figure in inputs to *K* or propositions which are outputs of *K*. You might also do so when evaluating beliefs to which the links in question are germane, whether they be your own or those of others. Let us say that if you have the capacity to take into account the existence of an inferential link in these and kindred ways then you are *sensitive* to that inferential link. What we need for our account of governance is the idea that if you are governed by a pattern *K* then inferential links instantiating K satisfy the condition that you are sensitive to these links. If you are thus sensitive then there is a sense in which you are guided by the pattern even though you may have no thoughts about it.[7]

Summing up the discussion we may think of being governed by a pattern of inference as a matter of having habits of belief management such as those described and sensitivity to inferential links instantiating the pattern. This view allows both for beliefs which are formed or abandoned unreflectively and also for beliefs which are formed or abandoned as a result of chains of reasoning in which the existence of certain inferential links is

[6] Rips (1988) surveys recent psychological work on deductive inference. As Rips notes there is ample evidence that there are simple but invalid inferences which a large percentage of people appear to regard as valid. It seems to me doubtful that this testifies to lack of competence in grasping the inferential role of the relevant concepts. Competence relates to patterns by which concepts are individuated. The inference patterns which create the problem may not fall into this class.

[7] Sellars (1954) is an important early discussion of the idea of pattern-governed behaviour.

explicitly taken into account. Our Competence condition requires that if *A*'s belief that *p* derives justification from his beliefs that *q*, *r*, . . . then *A*'s believing that *p* because he believes that *q*, *r*, . . . is an exercise of competence in relation to the relevant patterns of inference. We can now be more specific about what this means. To be competent in relation to a pattern of inference is to be governed by it. The Competence condition will be fulfilled if *A*'s belief that *p* is formed or maintained as a result of the exercise of appropriate habits of belief management or as a result of a chain of reasoning in which he has satisfied himself that an appropriate series of inferential links obtains.

Note that the Competence condition does not demand that a belief to the effect that *q*, *r*, . . . is an unconditional reason for *p* should figure as a component in the basis of the belief that *p*. This is just as well since it would lead to an infinite regress of the Achilles and the Tortoise type.[8] But we should not go to the extreme of supposing that such a belief can never have a role in the management of our beliefs. Nor should we get cold feet over the idea that such beliefs can contribute to the justification of other beliefs. We are led into a vicious regress only if we assume that if a belief that *p* depends for its justification on beliefs that *q*, *r*, . . . then the belief that *q*, *r*, . . . constitute a reason for *p must* form part of the basis of the belief that *p*. No such assumption is made on the account I have offered.

2.3. *The Basis*

Thus far we have a Basing condition, a Rational Connection condition and a Competence condition. The last condition I shall consider is a *Basis condition*. The formulation I shall give is rather vague, for reasons which will emerge.

JUS4 *A*'s belief that *p* derives its justification from his beliefs

[8] For a suggestive discussion, see Stroud (1979). Stroud asks, 'What is involved in someone's believing something on the basis of something else he knows or believes?'. He comments, 'This is not simply a question about the relation between the propositions the person believes' (pp. 184–5). That is why for justifiably basing a belief on others we need a Basing condition, interpreted in causal terms, and a Competence condition, as well as a Rational Connection condition. Winters (1983) is also germane.

> that *q*, *r*, . . . only if *A* legitimately takes it for granted that *q*, *r*, ...

The crucial question raised by *JUS4* is, of course, 'What is required in order that we may legitimately take it for granted that some proposition is true?' An obvious suggestion is that what is required is that we be justified in believing the proposition in question. However, this raises problems. In the usual sense, to be justified in believing that *p* implies believing that *p* on adequate grounds, and that comes to the same thing as being derivatively justified in believing that *p*. I shall argue later (Chapters 3 and 6) that we may legitimately take for granted many propositions which we are not justified in believing in the usual sense. In this respect I agree with those who have thought that there are groundless yet legitimately held beliefs.[9]

Notwithstanding these remarks it is clear that sometimes at least the legitimacy of taking for granted a proposition depends on its being justified itself. This suffices to generate the familiar problem about whether, and if so how, chains of derived justification terminate. I shall defer consideration of this problem until Chapter 6, where I shall also explore the issue of legitimately groundless belief. Henceforth I shall assume that justified belief is always in some sense derivatively justified. In Chapter 4 I shall argue that some beliefs derive their justification in part from current experience.

2.4. *Unconditional Inconclusive Reasons*

In this section I shall introduce a particular kind of reason and consider how such reasons relate to evidence.

We saw that *q*, *r*, . . . is an unconditional reason for *p* if *p* may be inferred from *q*, *r*, . . . without further ado, that is, without relying on further premisses besides *q*, *r*, ... The inference need not be deductively valid. In deductive cases the unconditional reason may be said to be a *conclusive* reason for the proposition for which it is a reason, but the notion of a conclusive reason should not be conflated with that of an

[9] I take it that this view is expressed in Wittgenstein (1969). See also Michael Williams (1977) and Malcolm (1977).

unconditional reason. *q*, *r*, . . . is a conclusive reason for *p*, in the sense intended here, if and only if it is not possible that *q*, *r*, . . . are all true and *p* false. I shall argue that some unconditional reasons are inconclusive.[10] But first we need to look at the notion of evidence.

Evidence for a hypothesis raises the chance that the hypothesis is true. As we ordinarily think of it evidence consists in facts. For example, the fact that the telephone extension cable has been cleanly severed is evidence that someone has been interfering with it. However, I shall follow the common practice of thinking of evidence as consisting in propositions. Thus I shall speak of proposition *e* as evidence for hypothesis *h*. If *e* is evidence for *h* then *e*'s being true constitutes evidence, in the more familiar sense, for *h*. To keep jargon to a minimum I shall use the term 'evidence' in both the familiar and the somewhat more specialized sense, leaving it to the context to indicate which is meant.

Sometimes *e* is evidence for *h* in a sense which implies that if *e* were true *h* would be true. In such cases I shall say that *e* is *infallible evidence* for *h*. Infallible evidence is the strongest there is. Often we are concerned with cases in which although *e*'s being true increases the chance that *h* is true, none the less *h* might be false even if *e* were true. In such cases I shall say that *e* is *fallible evidence* for *h*.[11] I shall concentrate on a type of case in which *e* and *h* each concern distinct token events or states of affairs. For example, that there are tracks of a certain type on a path might be evidence that deer have recently passed along that path. In the spirit of Hume, I shall take it that if this is so then the occurrence of tracks of that type on a path is a reliable indicator that deer have recently passed along it. Where the reliability is perfect we have an infallible evidential link, and where it is imperfect we have a fallible evidential link. Obviously fallible evidence admits of degrees. To simplify the discussion I shall confine my attention to cases of fallible evidence in which *e* raises to a high degree the chance that *h* is

[10] Note that sometimes the term 'conclusive' is used with a sense close to that of my 'unconditional'.

[11] The distinction between infallible and fallible evidence corresponds to Robert Nozick's distinction between strong and weak evidence. See Nozick (1981). I reserve the terms 'strong' and 'weak' for other purposes. See below.

true and in which therefore *e*'s being true would create a strong presumption in favour of *h*. These are cases in which *e* is *strong fallible evidence* for *h*.

At least in the type of case considered in this chapter the link between evidence and hypothesis is contingent.[12] Even in these cases, there is an important connection between *e*, the proposition that *e* is evidence of *h*, and *h*. For *e* and the proposition that *e* is evidence for *h* are components of an unconditional reason for *h*. It will emerge in the next section that this makes the connection just mentioned conceptual in a sense to be explained. But it is important to bear in mind that the evidential link itself, in the cases under consideration, is contingent and there need be no conceptual connection linking the propositions between which it holds.

I assume that on seeing that there are fresh-looking deer tracks on a path you might justifiably conclude that deer of a certain species have passed by recently. In that case some unconditional reason must be reflected in the basis of your belief. What sort of unconditional reason would fit the bill? Obviously, a component in such a reason could be the proposition that there are tracks of such-and-such a type on the path, but this by itself would be, at best, only a conditional reason for thinking that the deer have passed. An appropriate further premiss would be that there being tracks of the type in question on the path is infallible evidence of the recent passage of the deer. But you might be justified in concluding that these deer have passed even if you are not in a position to take it for granted that such an evidential link holds. You may know that there is another species of deer which is rare and not often seen in the area, and which also produces tracks like those on the path. Call deer in the first species *A*-deer and deer in the rare species *B*-deer. Tracks of the relevant type might occur even if no *A*-deer have passed. However, though you may not legitimately take it for granted that the occurrence of the tracks on the path is infallible evidence of the recent passage of *A*-deer

[12] I agree thus far with Nozick (1981). However, I differ radically from Nozick on the matter of how evidence bears on the justification of beliefs. Nozick defends a reliability theory of justification. At various points throughout the present work I contrast my own view of justification with reliability theories. See, in particular, 4.1. On the idea that there are non-contingent evidential links, see 4.3.

it could be that you may legitimately take it for granted that their occurrence is strong fallible evidence of the recent passage of *A*-deer.

Let *P* be the proposition that there are fresh-looking tracks of the relevant type on the path and *Q* the proposition that *A*-deer have recently passed by. To arrive at an appropriate unconditional reason for *Q* it might be suggested that we supplement *P* with *R*, the proposition that *P* is strong fallible evidence for *Q*. People who are not philosophers do not, by and large, speak of strong fallible evidence in the relevant sense and in so many words, but they speak in ways which show that they have a grasp of some such concept. We can imagine that those who know about animal tracks will speak of the occurrence of tracks of the type found on the path as a pretty sure sign that *A*-deer have passed by, while recognizing that just occasionally the tracks have been or could well have been produced by *B*-deer. Still, the amended proposal will not do. If you know that *B*-deer, though rare, have been in the area you could not justifiably conclude that *A*-deer have passed. For all you know the tracks might have been produced by the *B*-deer.

The problem is that the existence of strong though fallible evidence for *Q* is compatible with there being alternatives to *Q*, that is to say, hypotheses which account for the evidence without invoking *Q*. It seems that you must be in a position to discount these alternatives and that means being in a position to suppose that they do not provide the true explanation of the evidence.[13] Thus, knowing that *B*-deer produce tracks just like those on the path you must be in a position to take it for granted that they did not produce *these* tracks. Suppose we amend our account so that *P*, *R*, and the proposition that no alternative to *Q* is the true explanation of the evidence, together constitute an unconditional reason for *Q*. This seems to be along the right lines, but it raises a problem. There are countless alternatives to *Q*, including some which are outlandish, for instance that some crazy deer track forger, or a Martian antelope with feet just like *A*-deer, has been passing by, or that a Cartesian demon has been at

[13] I say *true* explanation simply to allow for explanations which do not spell out the actual reason why the phenomenon in question occurred. One could just as well speak of explanations (my true explanations) vs. merely putative explanations.

work. So we are faced with two related problems. First, it might seem that, short of having infallible evidence for *Q*, we will not be in a position to eliminate all the alternatives. But we were supposed to be considering a case of fallible evidence. Secondly, it seems absurd to suppose that we need to enquire into outlandish possibilities.

To see our way out of this problem we need the notion of a live alternative to *Q*. The live alternatives to *Q* are, roughly speaking, alternatives to *Q* which might well provide the true explanation of the evidence.[14] That *B*-deer have passed along the tracks recently might be a live alternative in the world of our example. That a crazy track forger has been at work would not be a live alternative to *Q*, if that world is anything like ours. Nor would the hypothesis that a Cartesian demon has been out to deceive us. Which alternatives we regard as live will depend on the prevailing background picture of the workings of the world for that will include presuppositions about what might and might not be the case. If you are to be in a position to conclude that *Q* is true you must be in a position to reject the view that any live alternative to *Q* is the true explanation of the evidence. This will be so only if you may take it for granted that there is a limited range of such alternatives, but we often are in this position. Now if you are in a position to reject the view that any live alternative to *Q* is the true explanation of the evidence, then, since all other alternatives may be ignored, you are in a position to reject the view that *P* is explained by some alternative to *Q*.

Taking these ideas into account, let *S* be the proposition that no alternative to *Q* provides a true explanation of the evidence. The amended proposal is that *P*, *R*, and *S* constitute an unconditional reason for *Q*.[15] Unfortunately, even this will not do. Granted *P*, *R*, and *S* you may none the less know of evidence that *Q* is false which outweighs the evidence supplied by the tracks. A team of round-the-clock observers may report that no *A*-deer have passed along the path recently. To deal with this it is not enough merely to require that you lack a reason for

[14] One may think of the live alternatives as being true in nearby possible worlds.

[15] Note that this is still an inconclusive reason in my sense. It is not logically necessary that there be a true explanation of the evidence.

thinking that there is overriding evidence for not-*Q*, in the sense which implies believing something which is a reason for thinking there is such evidence. Maybe such evidence is staring you in the face and you just ignore it. It seems that you need to be in a position to take it for granted that there is none. However, this might be thought to present a problem. Suppose that the path in question has characteristics to which *A*-deer are strangely averse. That the path has these characteristics might be strong fallible evidence that no *A*-deer have walked along it, yet we may not be able to detect the evidence or able to recognize it as evidence. This might suggest that since it is always logically possible for there to be evidence of this sort, we can never be assured that there is none. Yet if no one could be expected to have any inkling of the evidential link between the characteristics in question and the absence of *A*-deer, the fact that they are present would surely not militate against the legitimacy of concluding that *Q* is true. The problem is real only if we can never legitimately take for granted that there is no evidence for not-*Q*, and that has not been shown. Where the possibilities we need to take seriously—the live possibilities—are limited we can be in a position to take for granted that no such evidence exists. Let *T* be the proposition that there is no overriding evidence for not-*Q*. The proposal, finally amended, is that *P*, *R*, *S*, *T* constitute an unconditional reason for *Q*.

To suggest that a reason such as this may figure in the basis of a person's belief that *Q* is true, in the way required by our conditions on derived justification, is not to imply that the person must make conscious judgements with *P*, *R*, *S*, or *T* as contents. An experienced gamekeeper might see that the tracks in question are on the path without thinking to himself that the tracks are there. And he might justifiably come to believe that *A*-deer have passed without thinking to himself that the tracks are evidence of the recent passage of *A*-deer and without giving any thought to live alternatives to *Q* or counter-evidence to *Q* falling within the range of live possibilities. Such a person is likely to have a standing belief that the tracks are a pretty sure sign of *A*-deer and the circumstances may be such that the existence of alternatives or counter-evidence may be tacitly discounted without enquiry. It might be known, for instance, that for some time the *B*-deer have been fenced in somewhere else on the estate and there might be nothing which it would be reasonable to reckon as possible counter-evidence to *Q*.

If there is either an alternative to *h*, relative to evidence *e*, which is the true explanation of *e*, or if there is overriding evidence for not-*h*, I shall say that there are countervailing facts with respect to the presumption that *e* gives to *h*, or, more briefly, with respect to *h*. Countervailing facts with respect to *h* are facts which undermine the presumption in favour of *h* provided by *e*.

We saw that unconditional reasons are underwritten by patterns of inference. The unconditional reason we have arrived at would be underwritten by some such pattern as the following:

> *e*
> *e* is strong fallible evidence of *h*
> There are no countervailing facts with respect to *h*
> ———————————————————
> *h*

The kind of reason which this pattern underwrites is unconditional yet inconclusive. We acknowledge such reasons when we make inferences from evidence. The idea is that you may infer *Q* from *P*, *R*, *S*, *T* without further ado, yet clearly it is possible that *Q* is false even when these other propositions are true.[16] In being governed by the inference pattern which underwrites this reason we are not committed to supposing of any input to the pattern and its corresponding output that if the input is true the corresponding output is. However, we are committed to supposing of any input *I* to the pattern and corresponding output *O* something which is tantamount to the claim that *I* constitutes an unconditional reason for *O*. This is part of what is involved in being governed by the pattern. A presupposition of such a commitment is that the inference pattern in question is, though not truth-preserving, at least truth-conducive. That is to say, roughly, that inferences (in the psychological sense) made from true inputs to corresponding outputs would more often than not yield true conclusions. But that need not be a thought

[16] On the idea that *p* can be a reason for *q* even when it is not true that if *p* then *q*, see Thomson (1965), pp. 295 ff., and Stroud (1979).

that we frame for ourselves any more than in being governed by the deductive inference pattern *modus ponens* we need frame for ourselves the thought that it is truth-preserving.

In Chapter 3 I shall be concerned with a kind of inference from evidence which has caused much consternation among philosophers, namely inference from behaviour to the occurrence of pain. The type of reason considered in this section will provide us with a model with which to compare and contrast the type of reason related to these inferences. The topic is of interest on its own account. However, the reader who is resistant to being led up side-paths should bear in mind that the discussion of Chapter 3 will have direct relevance to the major theme of Chapter 4, the question whether experiences contribute to the justification of beliefs.

2.5. *Concepts and Inextricability*

In 2.2 I made use of the idea that mastery of a concept involves a grasp of its inferential role. In this section I shall explore this idea more fully. As a first approximation we may say that concepts are individuated by means of patterns of legitimate inference and that to possess, and thus have mastery of, a concept is to be governed by the patterns by which it is individuated. The claim about individuation is that concept *C* will be identical with concept *C*' if and only if *C* and *C*' are each, as we might say, exhibited by the same patterns of inference. What is it for a concept to be exhibited by a pattern of inference? An instance of the relation in question is that in which the concept of a garage stands to the pattern which is formulated as follows:

$$\frac{X \text{ is a garage}}{X \text{ is a place for storing or replacing motor vehicles}}$$

A concept may be conceived abstractly as a package of patterns of legitimate inference. These patterns determine the inferential role of the concept—its contribution to the inferential powers of propositions in which it figures. Thus the patterns which exhibit a concept characterize its inferential role.

The general idea applies as much to logical concepts, such as those of conjunction, disjunction, negation, and conditionality, as it does to descriptive concepts. Indeed, it is in connection with logical concepts expressible in the formalized languages of logic that the idea has had its most sustained and systematic elaboration, though usually expressed in terms of principles or rules of inference.[17] The hope is that it extends to concepts, both logical and descriptive, expressible in natural languages too. In the case of first-order languages of logic the inferential role of logical concepts is in each case given by patterns of inference which introduce the concept, that is, yield conclusions containing the concept from premisses which may not contain the concept, and patterns of inference which eliminate the concept, that is, yield conclusions which may not contain the concept from premisses at least one of which contains the concept. Clearly, the notion of introduction and elimination patterns extends also to descriptive concepts. The pattern specified above in connection with the concept of a garage is an elimination pattern for that concept. It seems plausible that for each concept there must be introduction and elimination patterns which suffice to account for what can be inferred from propositions containing the concept and what propositions containing that concept can be inferred from. The discussion of the last section opens up the prospect of there being introduction and elimination patterns which underwrite unconditional yet inconclusive reasons. The pattern identified towards the end of the section may be conceived as an elimination pattern for the tandem concepts of strong fallible evidence for *h* and of countervailing facts with respect to *h*.

As I said above, to possess a concept is to be governed by the patterns of inference by which it is individuated. But it needs to be remembered that concepts are components of networks. To possess the concept of a garage you have to possess the concepts which are the ingredients of the complex concept of a place for storing or repairing motor vehicles. So if one is

[17] This idea is crucially important in Michael Dummett's philosophy of language. See Dummett (1981, 1978) on the grounds and consequences of assertions. For extensions of the idea and their relevance to epistemology, see Peacocke (1986). On the idea that epistemic norms are built into concepts, see Pollock (1987).

governed by the patterns which exhibit the concept of a garage one must also be governed by the patterns which exhibit those ingredient concepts.

There is a traditional view that concepts, as it were, generate conceptual truths. The present analytical framework accommodates this view since it allows that in virtue of possessing a concept one is committed to taking certain propositions to be true. Possessing any concept incurs a commitment to accepting a range of rational-connection propositions, that is, propositions to the effect that a series of propositions constitutes an unconditional reason for some other proposition. However, the paradigm cases of conceptual truths, such as, that a garage is a place for storing or repairing motor vehicles, are not of this type. They are simply propositions which are inferable, without any undischarged assumptions, using inference patterns which underwrite conclusive reasons. Whenever any such proposition is true a corresponding rational-connection proposition is true, and vice versa. In the case of the garage example just given the corresponding rational-connection proposition is to the effect that something's being a garage is a conclusive reason for thinking it is a place for storing or repairing motor vehicles. Rational-connection propositions relating to inconclusive reasons, such as that which figures in the deer track example, do not correspond to traditional conceptual truths.

There is a vexing issue which threatens to undermine the general approach to concepts which I have been defending. According to that approach the concept of a mother-in-law, for example, is exhibited by the following patterns of inference:

$$\frac{A \text{ is the mother-in-law of } B}{A \text{ is the mother of the spouse of } B}$$

$$\frac{A \text{ is the mother of the spouse of } B}{A \text{ is the mother-in-law of } B}$$

If this is right then the proposition that Mary is the mother of Linda's spouse can be inferred from the proposition that Mary is the mother-in-law of Linda without further ado. By contrast the proposition that Mary has a tendency to resent Linda cannot be inferred from the proposition that Mary is the mother-in-law of Linda without further ado, though there are assumptions which together with the latter proposition would yield the former. This last point reflects the fact that the pattern of inference formulated as follows is not concept-exhibiting:

$$\frac{A \text{ is the mother-in-law of } B}{A \text{ has a tendency to resent } B}$$

This seems intuitively right, but there is a line of thought which casts doubt on whether we have any clear notion of what makes a pattern of inference concept-exhibiting. So far as descriptive concepts are concerned the idea is that there is no way of extricating from among those inferences made to or from propositions incorporating a concept *C* some special class of inferences instantiating patterns which exhibit *C*, as opposed to mere assumptions about instances of *C*. This is a variant of what Michael Dummett has called the *Inextricability thesis*.[18]

One could be forgiven for thinking that there is an obvious objection to the inextricability thesis. If the thesis were correct then there would be no distinction between inferring *p* from *q* without further ado and inferring *p* from *q* together with some other assumptions. There clearly is such a distinction, so the inextricability thesis is not correct. But while this response is on the side of the angels it will not do as it stands. The defender of the inextricability thesis will suggest that the distinction between inferring *p* from *q* without further ado and inferring *p* from *q* together with further assumptions is problematic. Returning to our example, the suggestion would be that both the inference from

Mary is the mother-in-law of Linda

to

Mary is the mother of Linda's spouse

[18] See Dummett (1978).

and that from

Mary is the mother-in-law of Linda

to

Mary has a tendency to resent Linda

rely on assumptions. In the first case the assumption is that, for any *a* and *b*, if *a* is the mother-in-law of *b* then *a* is the mother of the spouse of *b*, and in the second case the assumption is that, for any *a* and *b*, if *a* is the mother-in-law of *b* then *a* has a tendency to resent *b*. We might protest that the first of the propositions just mentioned is a straightforward conceptual truth, but the second is not. Again, I think this is right, but, again, it does not suffice to meet the challenge posed by the inextricability theorist, who will now suggest that the distinction between conceptual and non-conceptual truths is just as problematic as that between inferences which can be made without further ado and those which cannot.

At this point we may mount a counter-challenge to the inextricability theorist. Surely, on any view of the matter some conclusions follow from premisses without further ado. So there is nothing awry about the basic idea of conclusions following thus from premisses. The suggestion is that it is plausible to treat the first inference displayed above in this way but not the second. We have at least some inclination to suppose that whereas a further premiss is required for the second inference, none is required for the first. And this is linked to the plausible idea that if you grasp the concept of a mother-in-law you are committed to regarding Mary's being the mother-in-law of Linda as a conclusive reason for thinking that she is the mother of Linda's spouse, but you are not committed to regarding Mary's being the mother-in-law of Linda as a conclusive reason for thinking that Mary has a tendency to resent Linda.

There is a more and a less radical response which the inextricability theorist can make to this challenge. Both responses involve conceding that there is a sense in which some conclusions follow from premisses without further ado. The radical response is to suggest first, that the cases in which this is true are of inferences which hinge on purely logical operators, and secondly, that one can give an adequate account of these inferences without relying on a theory of concepts or of concept-exhibiting inference patterns. This radical response is very much in the spirit of W. V. Quine's thought on these matters.[19] The less radical response takes over the first component of the radical response, concedes that inferences which hinge solely on logical operators instantiate concept-exhibiting patterns of inference, but claims that such inferences are unproblematic by contrast with those which allegedly instantiate patterns exhibiting descriptive concepts. Neither response is satisfying. There is reason to think that a theory of concepts, which includes an account of logical and descriptive concepts, is indispensable.

A series of reflections clearly set out by Gareth Evans shows why.[20] Evans writes:

> [T]here must be a sense in which thoughts are structured. The thought that John is happy has something in common with the thought that Harry is happy, and the thought that John is happy has something in common with the thought that John is sad.[21]

Evans proposes to explain the sense in which thoughts are structured

> in terms of their being a complex of the exercise of several distinct conceptual *abilities*. Thus someone who thinks that John is happy and that Harry is happy exercises on two occasions the conceptual ability which we call 'possessing the concept of happiness'. And similarly someone who thinks that John is happy and that John is sad exercises on two occasions a single ability, the ability to think of, or think about, John.[22]

In the context of these passages Evans was especially concerned with the ability to think about individuals. I naturally want to focus on abilities linked to descriptive and logical concepts. Evans's point about structure seems to me to put beyond reasonable doubt the proposition that conceptual abilities must be reckoned with in any adequate account of thought and belief. Furthermore, our theory of how concepts, considered abstractly, are individuated must reflect those conceptual abilities

[19] The classic source is Quine's 'Two Dogmas of Empiricism' in Quine (1961). For trenchant criticisms of Quine's attempt to elucidate the notion of logical truth without recourse to a theory of concepts or propositions, see Strawson (1957). To my way of thinking Strawson's criticisms have never been adequately met.

[20] See Evans (1982). [21] Ibid., p. 100. [22] Ibid., p. 101.

which our modes of belief management and evaluation make it reasonable to suppose we have. If this is correct then there really ought to be no dispute over whether we need a theory of concepts, though there may be, and, of course, there are, disputes over how concepts are individuated.

We can hardly avoid regarding the use of logical expressions as reflecting conceptual abilities too. For when you think that John is happy and Harry is happy and then think that Bill is sad and Fred is sad, you exercise on each occasion an ability which stands to your use of the connective 'and' as the ability which consists in your possessing the concept of being happy stands to your use of the term 'happy'. Moreover, the first of these abilities is sufficiently analogous to the second to warrant being regarded as conceptual. It is a further step to the particular view of concepts which I have espoused, but an obvious point in favour of that view is that it yields a plausible account of conceptual capacities. Conceptual capacities are to be understood in terms of inferential competence.[23]

These considerations make both the radical and the less radical responses to the counter-challenge mounted a few paragraphs back extremely unappealing. A plausible account of logical particles will regard them as expressing logical concepts, just as a plausible account of descriptive expressions will conceive of them as expressing descriptive concepts. This line of thought is reinforced by the pleasing prospect of a uniform treatment of the individuation of concepts in terms of patterns of inference. However, the inextricability theorist will now challenge us to explain why we are so sure that whereas the proposition that Mary is the mother of the spouse of Linda follows from the proposition that Mary is the mother-in-law of Linda without further ado, the proposition that Mary has a tendency to resent Linda does not. The highly general considerations suggested by Evans's points about structure do not themselves cast light on this matter.

If there really is a difference between the two inferences at the abstract inter-propositional level this ought to reflect a difference at the level of individual psychology, the point being that

[23] Geach (1957) is an instructive earlier discussion of conceptual capacities and the structure of judgements. More recently, Campbell (1986) illuminatingly explores the links between structure, concepts, and inference.

if our thinking is governed by patterns of inference then descriptions of abstract inferential links must reflect facts about how people as a matter of fact think. The trouble is that if Linda, say, has a stable belief that all mothers-in-law have a tendency to resent the spouses of their offspring, then it will be true of her that she is disposed to infer that *A* has a tendency to resent *B* from the fact that *A* is the mother-in-law of *B*, just as she is disposed to infer that *A* is the mother of the spouse of *B* from the fact that *A* is the mother-in-law of *B*. So where is the required difference at the psychological level?

This train of thought assumes too simple a view of the psychology of concept possession. If the inference from 'Mary is the mother-in-law of Linda' to 'Mary has a tendency to resent Linda' instantiates a concept-exhibiting pattern then people who possess the concept of a mother-in-law will count *A*'s being the mother-in-law of *B* as a conclusive reason for thinking that *A* has a tendency to resent *B*. To meet that condition Linda must take the question whether *A* has a tendency to resent *B* as being settled by the mere fact that *A* is the mother-in-law of *B*. This will not be true of Linda if her use of the term 'mother-in-law' is the same as ours. For in that case she will be prepared to regard the claim that mothers-in-law have a tendency to resent the spouses of their offspring as an assumption, which even if widely held is in principle capable of refutation. And if that is so then the fact that *A* is the mother-in-law of *B* does not suffice to settle that *A* has a tendency to resent *B*.

These considerations lend substance to the claim that there is a difference between employing our familiar concept of a mother-in-law and employing a concept which would sanction the inference from 'Mary is the mother-in-law of Linda' to 'Mary has a tendency to resent Linda'. They would not convince Quine since they make free use of assumptions about propositional attitudes. Quine argues that if we adopt the standpoint of radical translators and try to recapitulate how we might arrive at the beliefs of others from their dispositions to verbal behaviour alone, we shall soon find that no unique scheme of propositional attitudes is demanded by the dispositions. Since in Quine's view such facts as there might be about which attitudes people have would have to supervene upon facts about verbal dispositions, it follows that there is no fact of the matter as to which attitudes people really have. Thus translation is indeterminate.[24]

I think that the route to the indeterminacy thesis is highly suspect, though it is not to be dismissed in a few paragraphs. The point I want to stress now is this: We do in fact conceive of one another as having specifiable propositional attitudes and in doing so tacitly discern certain structures in the contents of these attitudes which reflect the inferential roles of their ingredients. The very notion of there being alternative translation schemes matching alternative propositional attitude schemes presupposes that one and the same sentence admits of readings in terms of different structured contents. The view of concepts which I have been defending is simply part of a story about what differences in structure are. It is a story which links abstract differences in structure to concrete differences in competence. An effective challenge to Quine's scepticism will have to rely on some such view.[25]

[24] See Quine (1960). An excellent recent discussion of the issues is contained in Hookway (1988).

[25] For a discussion along somewhat similar lines, see Hookway (1988).

3

Reasons, Justification, and Evidence II

3.1. *Evidence of Pain*

In Chapter 2 the concept of an unconditional inconclusive reason was introduced in relation to the example of the deer tracks. The question to be considered now is whether the reasons we rely on when we ascribe pain to others have essentially the same structure as the reason discerned in that example. The discussion, when taken together with that of the previous chapter, will take us closer to our exploration of whether, and if so how, sensory experiences contribute to the justification of beliefs.

On the face of it a positive answer to our question seems to be in order, for the occurrence of pain behaviour of various kinds seems to stand to the occurrence of pain as the occurrence of the deer tracks stood to the recent passage of deer. Let us focus on a particular kind of pain behaviour, namely wincing in response to pressure on some area of the body. Such behaviour is a highly reliable, though not an infallible, indicator that the subject is in pain. So we have a strong fallible evidential link akin to that in the deer case. We also have a conception of what would count as countervailing facts with respect to the hypothesis that the subject is in pain. There may be live alternatives to that hypothesis. For example, it might emerge that the subject is mentally unbalanced and has a history of wasting people's time by feigning pain. In that case the hypothesis that on the occasion in question the subject is feigning pain would be a live alternative to the hypothesis that he is in pain. Could there be, as in the deer case, evidence that the subject is not in pain in circumstances in which he realistically winces in response to pressure? Examples are difficult to find. The subject could always tell us that he is not in pain, but it seems implausible that such evidence would outweigh the evidence that the subject is in pain provided by his continuing to wince in a manner which shows all the signs of being spontaneous. We need something which would override the evidence that the subject is in pain. Suppose that there is a well-established theory correlating and explaining the correlation between pain and some type of physiological state. In that event, perhaps overriding evidence that the subject is not in pain would be provided by the fact that he showed no signs of being in the appropriate state. On the other hand, really convincing wincing might reasonably make us wonder whether the background theory can be right. No matter; if there were overriding evidence that the subject is not in pain that would amount to a countervailing fact with respect to the subject's being in pain.

Despite the analogies, there is a well-known line of thought according to which the pain case is crucially different from the deer case. It goes as follows. In the deer case, whether the occurrence of the tracks constitutes strong fallible evidence for the recent passage of deer is a contingent matter admitting straightforward empirical confirmation or disconfirmation. By contrast, according to this line of thought, it is a necessary truth that a subject's wincing in response to pressure constitutes strong fallible evidence that the subject is in pain, and the existence of this evidential link is not something which we can confirm or disconfirm empirically. Both of these points are captured by the claim that wincing in response to pressure is a *criterion* rather than merely a *symptom* of pain. According to the criterion theory, as I shall call it, the peculiar character of the evidential link between various kinds of pain behaviour and pain is supposed to be explained by the fact that it is a conceptual truth that these behaviours are strong fallible evidence of pain. Given the traditional view of concepts which this line of thought presupposes it follows that the evidential link holds necessarily and that the grounds for thinking that it holds are not empirical.[1]

[1] Remarks of Wittgenstein provide the inspiration for the criterion theory. See esp. Albritton (1959), but note the postscript added to the reprint in Pitcher (1968). Hacker (1972) discerns a criterion theory in Wittgenstein's remarks.

A major stumbling-block for the criterion theory is its claim that propositions to the effect that such-and-such a type of pain behaviour is evidence of pain are necessary truths. It should be stressed that the claim is not that, necessarily, if a person manifests pain behaviour of some specified type then that person is in pain. The criterion theorist is as anxious as I am to allow for the possibility that a subject should manifest pain behaviour and not be in pain.[2] The claim is only that it is a necessary truth that a person's manifesting pain behaviour of some type is strong fallible evidence that that person is in pain. Still, it is difficult to see what compels us to accept this central claim.

The very same behaviours which are usually caused by pain could equally be caused by other conditions. It seems to be a contingent fact concerning any particular type of pain behaviour that it is *usually* caused by pain rather than by something else. It could be that people for some obscure reason start to wince in response to pressure on many occasions when they are not in pain. So it could turn out that on most occasions when people react in this way they are not actually in pain. In that case, wincing in response to pressure would no longer reliably indicate pain, and thus would no longer be strong fallible evidence of pain, although it would still be true that people in pain commonly manifest that type of behaviour.

On the other hand, the criterion theory seems to be right in according a special role to the assumption that wincing in response to pressure is evidence of pain. We do not in fact take

Lycan (1971) is a useful survey. Wright (1987) contains important recent discussions. McDowell (1982) is critical of attempts to read a criterion theory on 'traditional' lines into Wittgenstein. In the text I have particularly in mind the theory which informed Shoemaker (1963). The following passage from that work is crucial: 'For present purposes we may characterise the criteria for the truth of a judgment as those states of affairs that are (whose existence would be) direct non-inductive evidence in favour of the truth of the judgment. A test of whether something is one of the criteria for the truth of judgments of a certain kind is whether it is conceivable that we might discover empirically that it is not or that it has ceased to be, evidence in favor of the truth of such judgments. If it is evidence, and it is not conceivable that it could be discovered not to be (or no longer to be) evidence, then it is one of the criteria. If so-and-so's being the case is a criterion for the truth of a judgment of Φ-identity, the assertion that it is evidence in favor of the truth of the judgment is necessarily (logically) rather than contingently (empirically) true' (pp. 3–4).

[2] McDowell (1982) appears to be an exception. I discuss this work in 3.4.

that assumption to be true because we have empirical confirmation for it. Rather it seems to be something which we come tacitly to accept as we learn how to tell when people, including ourselves, are in pain. Our problem is to do justice to the special role of the assumption while allowing that it is contingent.

3.2. *An Alternative to the Criterion Theory*

Let *P* be the proposition that Tom winces when pressure is applied to his abdomen, *Q* the proposition that Tom has a pain in his abdomen. Notwithstanding the remarks of the last section it seems plausible that, in parallel with the deer case, *Q* is inferable without further ado from *P* together with the proposition *R*, that *P* is strong fallible evidence for *Q*, and the proposition *S*, that there are no countervailing facts with respect to *Q*. The problem we face is how to do justice to the special status of *R*, but the fact that that is our problem does nothing to undermine the idea that the pain case has the inferential structure shown.

It is indisputable that our concept of pain is a concept of a state which expresses itself in certain distinctive ways. We think of pain as a distressing or discomforting sensitivity located in some region of the body, which is apt to result in responses like wincing, or other signs of discomfort or distress relating to that region, either spontaneously or if the region is stimulated by tactile pressure or in certain other ways, and which is itself apt to be caused by injury or disease. This suggests that something like the following is an introduction pattern for the concept of having a pain in some region of the body. '*U*' stands in place of names or singular descriptions of regions of the body.

> *A* experiences a distressing or discomforting sensitivity in *U* of a type occurrences of which are apt to cause wincing or other manifestations of distress or discomfort, relating to *U*, either spontaneously or in response to appropriate stimulation of *U*, and are themselves apt to be caused by physical injury or disease.
>
> ---
>
> *A* has a pain in *U*.

The corresponding elimination pattern goes from the conclusion of this introduction pattern to its premiss. These patterns account for the intuition that it is built into our understanding of the notion of pain that pains are apt to manifest themselves in the familiar ways. But to be governed by these patterns does not commit one to holding that pain behaviours are strong fallible evidence of pain. So even if our concept of pain is individuated by these patterns the special role of *R* in our example is not thereby explained.

We do have a notion of what counts as a pretty sure sign of someone's being in pain and that notion, not surprisingly, covers those behaviours by which pain commonly manifests itself. But from the fact that a behaviour is among those by which pain manifests itself it by no means follows that it is a reliable indicator of pain. For it is logically possible that the very same behaviour should, as often as not, be caused by conditions other than pain. Nevertheless, we do in fact regard the familiar pain behaviours as evidence of pain. For instance, we accept, in effect, the general evidential proposition that wincing in response to stimulation of a region of the body is strong fallible evidence that the subject is in pain. *R* is just an instance of this general evidential proposition. The question is how our acceptance of *R* relates to our possession of the concept of pain.

It is surely significant that we do not accept *R*, or the general evidential proposition of which it is an instance, on empirical grounds. I think we can shed some light on the matter by considering other evidential propositions of which this is also true.

Scars are the traces of healed wounds, burns, or sores. Various kinds of scars have distinctive appearances. Think of the kind caused by cutting flesh with a sharp blade. The occurrence of such a mark on a region of the surface of a person's body is (at least strong fallible) evidence that the person has been cut with a sharp blade in that region. Here we have a general evidential proposition which is indisputably contingent. It could have been the case that marks of this type were as often as not caused by something other than cutting with a sharp blade. (Indeed, it could have been the case that as often as not such marks were not scars at all, in the usual sense of that term.) Yet although the evidential proposition in question is contingent, most of us, I suspect, do not believe it to be true on empirical grounds. Some of us may well have noted how the appearance of various scars correlates with various kinds of injury. But many of us come to think of various marks as signs for different types of injury, not through having observed numerous cuttings and burnings in the act, so to speak, but simply through having been taught that this sort of mark is usually caused by a cut and this other by a burn. In fact our practice of applying the concept of a scar depends on our assuming that the familiar scar-type marks are usually scars in the full sense which implies that they were caused by wounds, burns, or sores.

Now it is not part of our understanding of what it is to be a scar that the familiar scar-type marks are usually traces of wounds, burns, or sores. If a mark is a scar it is the trace of a wound, burn, or sore, and if a mark is such a trace it is a scar. But if it should come about and we should discover that scar-type marks start to be produced as often as not by something other than wounds, burns, or sores our understanding of what it is to be a scar would be unaffected. What would have to change, in that event, is a familiar mode of application of the concept of a scar. That mode of application is linked to a pattern of inference from evidence of the type examined in connection with the deer track example. It rests on a presupposition to the effect that a mark's having such-and-such an appearance is strong fallible evidence that it is a scar. But if we should come to think the presupposition false we would no longer be in a position to judge that a mark is a scar from its appearance. What this suggests, I think, is that we need to distinguish between possessing a concept and employing some particular mode of application of the concept. Possessing a concept does not entail employing every mode of application of the concept. A mode of application could cease to be employed with no corresponding change in the concept. Still, we learn prevailing modes of application as we learn to employ the concept. In the case in hand we learn to presuppose the general evidential proposition linking scar-type marks with scars as we learn to employ the concept of a scar in line with the familiar mode of application.

Let us consider another somewhat similar example before we

return to the concept of pain.[3] In common parlance a thing is punctured or said to have a puncture if it has a hole or slit caused by insertion of a sharp object. The concept is most frequently employed these days in connection with pneumatic tyres and inner tubes. In applying it we assume the general evidential proposition that the occurrence of a hole or slit in a tyre or inner tube is (at least strong fallible) evidence that it has been punctured. I confidently apply the concept of a puncture, assuming this evidential proposition to be true, yet without ever having actually seen a sharp object insert itself into a tyre. Like most other people I learned what a puncture is by being shown how to detect holes or slits in tyres or inner tubes, and through being told that these are (usually) punctures and thus caused by puncturing, the insertion of sharp objects like broken glass or nails. In parallel with the scar case, it is not part of our understanding of what a puncture is that holes or slits of the familiar puncture-types are indeed usually punctures, for our understanding of what a puncture is could remain the same even if it were to come about that these holes and slits are as often as not produced by something other than puncturing. Rubber products might for some reason develop highly localized weaknesses which result in small puncture-like slits or holes even in the absence of external damage. If we were to discover this to be so we would no longer be in a position to judge that a tyre has a puncture, in the original sense, from the fact that it has a small puncture-type hole or slit. So, again as in the scar case, our mode of applying the concept of a puncture would need to change since a general evidential proposition which the practice presupposes could no longer be relied on. Of course, we might well modify our concept of a puncture so that it covers any smallish hole or slit. The point is that abandoning the mode of application of the concept which we have been considering would not in itself show that we had modified the concept.

The pain case is similar to the two cases just considered in these respects: It is not part of our understanding of what pain is that familiar pain behaviours are evidence of pain. Our concept

[3] The example is adapted from Bernard Williams's 'Knowledge and Meaning in the Philosophy of Mind' which occurs in Williams (1973), pp. 127–35. See in particular pp. 132 ff.

of pain allows for the possibility that it should come about (or that it be true now) that some such behaviours are as often as not produced by something other than pain. However, if we were to discover this to be so our mode of applying the concept of pain would have to change for it rests on the assumption that pain behaviours are strong fallible evidence (a pretty sure sign) of pain. This assumption is not something which we accept on empirical grounds. Rather, it is something we learn tacitly to regard as true as we learn to apply the concept in line with the familiar mode of application.

We have then a number of cases in which there exists a stable practice of applying a concept which rests on the assumption of an evidential proposition. A feature of these cases is that people come to regard the relevant evidential proposition as true simply through learning to apply the concept in line with the prevailing mode of application and without regard to empirical or theoretical grounds. It may be that for some of these propositions there are or could be empirical or theoretical grounds for thinking them true. For others, such as those involved in ascriptions of pain, it may be problematic whether there are or could be grounds for thinking them true. But the important thing is that those who employ the concept in line with the prevailing mode of application learn to count such a proposition true.

In the light of the foregoing reflections it is useful to distinguish between a narrow and a broad sense of mastery of a concept. In the narrow sense, to master a concept is simply to possess it, which, to a first approximation, means to be governed by the inference patterns by which it is individuated (2.5). In the broader sense, mastering a concept involves everything which possession involves plus the mastery of any modes of application which though not entailed by possession nevertheless prevail among those for whom the concept has a use.

Nothing as yet has been said concerning our *right* to regard the evidential propositions under consideration as true. Our Basis condition *JUS4* (2.3) requires that if a belief derives its justification from others then the contents of the latter must be legitimately taken for granted. That taking for granted a proposition is fundamental for a conceptual practice does not in itself show that it is legitimate to do so. This brings us to large and controversial issues in the theory of knowledge. If the legitimate acceptance of a proposition requires that belief in the truth of the proposition should rest on adequate grounds—should be, in effect, derivatively justified—then, obviously, to accept a proposition on no grounds at all would not be legitimate. Many theorists would accept the antecedent of this conditional and detach the consequent. On the other hand, other philosophers have thought it can be legitimate to accept a proposition groundlessly.[4] I shall develop a view on this matter in Chapter 6. To anticipate: The view is that (*a*) once we take seriously the causal character of 'resting belief on grounds' it becomes clear that very many of our beliefs are groundless, yet (*b*) it is possible to make sense of the idea that groundless belief can be legitimate.

Central to the development of (*b*) is the idea of a *normative* proposition. Normative propositions are propositions which we learn to take for granted and treat as beyond dispute. Together with the concepts we employ they constitute a perspective on the world. According to the account given in 2.2 and 2.5 we possess a concept in so far as we are governed by the patterns of inference which exhibit the concept. There is a sense in which normative propositions may be said to govern our thinking too—we count them true and in managing our beliefs are sensitive to the fact that they are to be reckoned as beyond dispute. Thus if *P* governs our thinking we are prepared to enter it as an assumption in our reasonings without further ado. To have a competent grasp of a perspective requires not only a mastery of its constituent concepts but also a mastery of its constituent normative propositions, an ability, that is, to deploy those propositions as assumptions in managing our own beliefs and evaluating beliefs generally.

It is important to appreciate that not every proposition which we happen to accept is normative for us. The crucial thing about a normative proposition is that its acceptance is well entrenched and taking it to be true is not thought to require justification. As I shall have occasion to stress in Chapter 6, this does not mean that our attitude to such propositions is immune to revision.

[4] See n. 9 to Ch. 2.

Facts may emerge which force us to withdraw acceptance. Propositions only retain their status as normative so long as there is no manifest conflict between them and other propositions we feel compelled to accept.

It should not be thought that the normativity of a proposition is a reason for accepting it. Rather, the normativity of a proposition is just its governing our thinking. The fact that this involves being sensitive to the fact that it is to be reckoned as beyond dispute should not tempt us to look for some intrinsic feature of the proposition which makes it worthy to be reckoned in this way. There is nothing behind the shared practice of unquestioningly relying on the proposition which accounts for its having a normative role.

I want to suggest that the general evidential propositions we have been considering should be conceived as normative propositions and that they govern our thinking in the manner explained. This would account for our groundlessly accepting such propositions. If you were to reject *R* in our example, the proposition that Tom's wincing when pressure is applied to his abdomen is strong fallible evidence that he has a pain in his abdomen, you would be committed to rejecting the general evidential proposition of which it is an instance. But if the latter proposition is normative for you then you are committed to accepting it. The special status of *R* consists in the fact that it is an instance of a normative proposition the assumption of which lies behind our mode of applying the concept of pain to others. Criterion theorists were right to feel that *R* has a special status but wrong in the account which they gave of that status.

This is as far as I shall take the matter here, but it should be borne in mind that considerations which are germane to the proposed view will unfold in subsequent chapters.

3.3. *Mad Pain*

In the last section I adopted a broadly functionalist view of pain in so far as I held that pains are states which have a certain causal role: they are states which are apt to cause certain kinds of behaviour and are apt to be caused by certain sorts of circumstance. There are different ways of developing such a view. In this section I want to comment on a discussion of David Lewis which leads in directions to which I am not myself committed.[5]

Lewis's discussion begins with the following striking passage:

> There might be a strange man who sometimes feels pain, just as we do, but whose pain differs greatly from ours in its causes and effects. Our pain is typically caused by cuts, burns, pressure, and the like; his is caused by moderate exercise on an empty stomach. Our pain is generally distracting; his turns his mind to mathematics, facilitating concentration on that but distracting him from anything else. Intense pain has no tendency whatever to cause him to groan or writhe, but does cause him to cross his legs and snap his fingers. He is not in the least motivated to prevent pain or to get rid of it. In short, he feels pain but his pain does not at all occupy the typical causal role of pain.[6]

Lewis calls the pain which this person has 'mad pain'. He thinks that a credible theory of mind ought to allow for such a phenomenon. Since he also holds to a functionalist view of pain the problem, as he sees it, is to show that such a theory can cope with mad pain. My own intuitions on the matter are rather different. It seems to me that if the states of the madman which Lewis regards as pains are really so different in their causal role from the pain states of normal human beings then they are not pains. So it would worry me if my view of pain had as a consequence that mad pains are genuine pains.

My main concern, I suppose, is that mad pains appear not to be distressing or discomforting states. How else are we to interpret the fact that the subject has no tendency to avoid or prevent them and is not distracted by them in the usual way? Mad pains are not genuine pains unless they are distressing or discomforting, and we lose our grip on the notion that they are like this when their causal role in the mental/physical organization of the madman is quite different from the familiar causal role of pain.

How does Lewis accommodate mad pain? The trick is turned with the help of the notion of pain for a population. Human pain, that is pain for the population of humans, is a state which is said to occupy the causal role of pain for most human beings.

[5] See Lewis (1980), repr. in Lewis (1983). Page references are to the latter edn.
[6] Ibid., p. 122.

For a state to occupy this role all that is required is that the state is of a type such that typically among humans states of that type have the familiar causal role. The madman is just an exception. 'His state does not occupy the role of pain for a population comprising himself and his fellow madmen. But it does occupy that role for a more salient population—mankind at large.'[7]

My initial worry about this view was precisely that it makes it possible for pain in a given subject not typically to have for that subject the effects and causes prescribed by the familiar causal role of pain. So now the question is whether my view can block the possibility of this kind of divorce between the way pain functions in the organization of an individual and the usual causal role of pain.

The elucidation of the concept of pain given in the last section has it that pain is a state occurrences of which are apt to issue in certain behaviours either spontaneously or in response to stimuli and are apt to be caused by injury or disease. This might seem to amount to much the same as Lewis's view. However, the intended reading is that pain in a subject is a state occurrences of which *in that subject* are apt to have the familiar causes and effects. This rules out mad pain because mad pain is not apt to have the usual causes and effects. The reading is by no means *ad hoc*. It simply reflects the intuition which provoked the initial worry about mad pain and is consistent with a natural reading of 'apt'. To say that occurrences of a state are apt to have certain causes and effects might just mean that in most subjects most of the time such occurrences do have such causes and effects. (Lewis himself uses the term in this way.) But there is a stronger reading on which occurrences of a state would not be apt to have some behavioural effect (or other) in a range of such effects unless the subject had some tendency or inclination to produce an effect within the range. You may be stoically nursing an awful toothache for all the world as if nothing were troubling you, yet even then you will have at least a tendency to be distracted by the pain and to avoid putting pressure on the tooth. If you do none of these things it will be because you are exercising extraordinary self-control. In the normal course of events even mild pains have some behavioural effects. A

[7] Ibid., p. 127.

somewhat similar point applies to the causes of pain. In the strong sense, an occurrence of a state in a subject would not be apt to be caused by something (or other) in a range of causes, unless in the normal course of events in that subject it would be caused by something in the range. Mad pain is not genuine pain because it is not in the strong sense apt to have the usual effects and causes.

There is a temptation to think of pain in this way: We merely fix the reference of the name 'pain' when we say that pains are states which have a certain causal role. So having fixed it that 'pain' refers to states which have the familiar causal role, we can then go on to raise the question what pains are, as it were, in themselves, allowing, perhaps, if we are materialists, that what pains are in themselves may vary with different kinds of being. The idea is that while we have arranged that 'pain' refers to states of a certain type, we have not actually said which type.[8] Two developments are possible from here. Either we opt for specifying the types in neurophysiological terms or we opt for specifying them in terms of what it is like to have them, where the relevant typology is not given by causal role.

To my way of thinking this whole picture is deeply mistaken. It is wrong in the first place to think that we *merely fix* the reference of 'pain' when we say that pains have such-and-such a causal role for we have no notion of what makes a mental state the type it is other than in terms of causal roles. In fixing the reference via causal role we type the state. The further project which is supposed to be called for is not on. Lewis is far from supposing that we could specify the type of state which pains are in terms of what it is like to have them, where that is conceived other than in terms of causal role. But he seems to go for the neurophysiological option. In fact, his desire to allow for mad pain seems to spring less from pre-theoretical intuition than from the thought that the madman has pains because he is a human being and has just those neurophysiological states which in most of us have the usual causes and effects. This gives some content to the idea that mad pains are the same states as our pains. The trouble is that it gives no content to the thought that when he has mad pains the madman feels the same way we

[8] Compare the discussion of the typology of experience in 1.4.

do when we have pains. I do not think we can give content to such a thought unless pains are tied to something like the familiar causal role in the way I have suggested.

3.4. *Evidentialism with respect to Ascriptions of Pain*

My treatment of the ascription of pain to others shares with the criterion theory the idea that pain is ascribed to an individual on the basis of beliefs as to the occurrence of pain behaviours, where it is assumed that these behaviours can occur even though the individual is not in pain. Theories which incorporate this idea could be called *evidentialist* in that they treat behaviour as, in one way or another, evidence of a mental state. John McDowell has argued vigorously against such theories, though his principal target is the criterion theory as standardly conceived.[9]

McDowell thinks that the criterion theory relies on the following mistaken picture of our epistemological predicament.

> Judgements about other minds are, as a class, epistemologically problematic. Judgements about 'behaviour' and 'bodily' characteristics are, as a class, not epistemologically problematic; or at any rate, if they are, it is because of a different epistemological problem, which can be taken for these purposes to have been separately dealt with. The challenge is to explain how our unproblematic intake of 'behavioural' and 'bodily' information can adequately warrant our problematic judgements about other minds.[10]

In McDowell's view both the sceptic about other minds and the criterion theorist fasten on to this picture. They differ in that whereas the former argues that behavioural and bodily information cannot warrant judgements about the states of other minds, the latter tries to show how such information warrants such judgements. McDowell objects to the criterion theory, as I have done in 3.1, on the grounds that, contrary to what the theory holds, the ties between behaviour and bodily states on the one hand and mental states on the other are contingent.[11] He also objects to the picture which the criterion theory shares with scepticism. The picture, he writes,

[9] McDowell (1982). [10] Ibid., p. 468. [11] Ibid., p. 469.

involves a corpus of 'bodily' and 'behavioural' information, unproblematically available to us in a pictured cognitive predicament in which we are holding in suspense all attributions of psychological properties to others. . . . Human bodies, conceived as merely material objects, form the subject-matter of the supposed unproblematically available information. The idea is that they may subsequently turn out to be, in some more or less mysterious way, points of occupancy for psychological properties as well . . .[12]

McDowell is on to a point of great importance in this area. There is something radically mistaken about the idea that in practice we identify behaviour or bodily states as being of a sort that warrants ascriptions of mental states, yet in a manner which is compatible with our 'holding in suspense all attributions of psychological properties to others'. I differ from McDowell, however, in so far as I doubt that criterion theories or my own view need incorporate the mistaken notion. It has to be admitted that criterion theories have been offered as responses to scepticism and criterion theorists may have conceded too much to scepticism. Still, it is not clear that such theorists need be committed to the mistaken notion just mentioned. Criterion theorists, and evidentialists generally, certainly are committed to the idea that mental states can be justifiably ascribed (roughly speaking) on the basis of behaviour or bodily states identifiable independently of whether the subject is or is not in the mental state which the behaviour or bodily state provides a warrant for ascribing. My own approach shares this commitment, but is not thereby committed to the notion that our concepts of the relevant sorts of behaviour or bodily states permit the suspense of all attributions of psychological properties to others.

People can wince, writhe, and groan yet not be in pain. It does not follow that our wincing, writhing, and groaning are purely behavioural or bodily in a sense which leaves it an open question whether those who display these behaviours are subjects of mental states. I suspect that we learn what wincing is ostensively. We learn that it is that sort of reaction on the part of creatures like *these*, where *these* are creatures which we think of, and react to, as, like us, subjects of feelings, if not beliefs and other propositional attitudes. If this is correct then our concept of wincing applies to human beings and, by analogy with them,

12 McDowell (1982).

to other animals. The practice of applying the concept presupposes that the range of objects to which it applies are bearers of psychological properties, so there is no question of applying these concepts and suspending *all* attributions of psychological properties.

McDowell's own positive view is that we can come to know that someone is in pain on the basis of what they say and how they look. Yet the view is not evidentialist, for McDowell thinks that expressions of pain are 'directly available to experience'.[13] What this means is that the data on the basis of which we ascribe pain to a person do not merely constitute strong fallible evidence that the person is in pain; rather they constitute a manifestation of pain, in a sense which implies that the subject really is in pain. So although the person's manifesting pain is not quite the same as the person's being in pain, nevertheless, it does not fall short of the subject's being in pain in the way that pain behaviour does on my view or on the criterion theory as I have explained it. As McDowell sees it, there is a sense in which on these latter views knowledge that someone is in pain is inferential so that its 'content . . . is generated by a transformation of the content of some data'. By contrast, on McDowell's own view, as he neatly puts it, 'the content of the knowledge is simply presented in the data'.[14] McDowell favours this view at least in part because he wishes to avoid the picture mentioned above which he thinks criterion theorists share with sceptics. As we have seen, there are ways of avoiding that picture consistent with an evidentialist view. However, there is another element in the motivation of McDowell's position. He wishes to resist the idea that the appearance of being in a mental state like pain is a common factor in cases in which the subject is in pain and cases where this is not so, and this is tied up with his understanding of how manifestations of pain are directly available to experience. McDowell acknowledges, as he must, that our capacity to tell whether another is in pain is fallible, but he is anxious to resist the lure of the following argument.

> [S]ince there can be deceptive cases experientially indistinguishable from non-deceptive cases, one's experiential intake . . . must be the same in both kinds of case. In a deceptive case, one's experiential intake

[13] Ibid., p. 473. [14] Ibid.

must *ex hypothesi* fall short of the fact itself, in the sense of being consistent with there being no such fact. So that must be true, according to the argument, in a non-deceptive case too.[15]

McDowell thinks that allied to this line of thought is the idea that '[i]n a deceptive case, what is embraced within the scope of experience is an appearance that such-and-such is the case, falling short of the fact: a *mere* appearance' and so 'what is experienced in a non-deceptive case is a mere appearance as well'.[16] He wishes to oppose this with an alternative picture according to which the appearance that is presented in the non-deceptive cases 'is a matter of the fact itself being disclosed to the experiencer'. This being so, 'appearances are no longer conceived as in general intervening between the experiencing subject and the world'.[17]

With this last gloss, about appearances intervening between the experiencing subject and the world, McDowell again reads too much into the opponent's position, since the appearances in question, if we allow ourselves to speak in this way, are as much part of the world as pains are. That a person looks to be in pain is a thoroughly worldly state of affairs, not a fragment of any veil of appearance between subjects and their world.[18] But, important though it is, that point does not touch the nub of the issue which McDowell wants to tackle. This is, I take it, the suggestion that if the appearance of being in pain is common to the deceptive and non-deceptive cases, then it cannot be the case that manifestations of pain, conceived as occurring only in non-deceptive cases, are directly available to experience as McDowell thinks they are.

Needless to say, it all depends what you mean by 'directly available to experience'. McDowell's treatment of this notion is not overly systematic. It seems fairly clear though that something's being directly available to experience is to be contrasted with cases in which something is known to obtain through inference from something else. The view is that manifestations of pain can function as data for knowledge but, as we have seen, McDowell thinks that the knowledge that someone is in pain is

[15] McDowell (1982), p. 471. [16] Ibid., p. 472. [17] Ibid.

[18] It is worth recalling also the remarks in the Introduction about misleading conceptions of experience. Experiences do not form a veil between us and the world any more than appearances do.

not inferential, because 'the content of the knowledge is simply presented in the data'. Yet he seems to suggest[19] that the fact that someone is in pain need not itself be regarded as a candidate for being directly available to experience. In other words, McDowell blocks the inference from 'The fact that *p* is directly available to experience' and 'The fact that *p* presents the fact that *q*' to 'The fact that *q* is directly available to experience'. It is far from clear what systematic account of direct availability and of presenting could plausibly explain why this inference would be illegitimate. Rather than speculate about that matter I want to take a different tack.

McDowell is right in thinking that there is an important sense in which the knowledge that someone is in pain, gleaned from looking at that person's manifestations of pain, is not inferential. If inferential knowledge results from inference, in the sense of a chain of reasoning, then knowledge of the sort in question need not be inferential. While looking at a person who manifests pain we may acquire a mass of beliefs including the belief that the subject is in pain, the belief that the subject manifests pain, the belief that the subject is wincing as pressure is applied to the appropriate region, and many other beliefs besides having nothing to do with pain. There need be no question of having first acquired a belief that the subject is wincing, or displaying some other kind of behaviour which we think of as reliably indicative of pain, and then reflecting that since the subject displays the behaviour in question and since various auxiliary assumptions hold, the subject is in pain.

Notwithstanding the preceding remarks it is worth noting in passing that even if beliefs that people are in pain, gleaned from looking at them, are not, or not always, acquired through inference in the sense just mentioned, it may yet be true, and surely is in fact true, that we can and do reason to the conclusion that people are in pain from information about the way they behave, where this latter information is available to us other than through our having perceived the people themselves. For instance, we might be told simply that a man was clutching his head after having been beaten with a wooden club. From this and other information obtained at second hand about

[19] McDowell (1982), p. 473.

the context we might legitimately infer that the man was in pain. We would thus have a chain of reasoning which would lend itself to some kind of evidentialist analysis.

Still, there is no getting round the fact that McDowell is concerned with perceptual cases and with regard to these at least finds the evidentialist approach to be wanting. He finds that approach wanting, I suspect, because he tacitly assumes that abstract inferential structures do not bear on the justification of a belief unless the belief results from a chain of reasoning. But this assumption is false. The particular evidentialist approach which I presented in 3.2 involved an analysis of a kind of abstract reason-for-thinking that someone is in pain, a reason which incorporated a proposition to the effect that the subject displays pain behaviour of some type. This kind of reason can be implicated in the justification of a belief, in the way indicated in *JUS2'* of 2.2, even where the belief does not result from a chain of reasoning.

We need to recall here that a belief can be based on other beliefs even if it is not brought about by these beliefs. Suppose you acquire, in a way which essentially involves perception, the belief that Tom is in pain, the belief that he winces when pressure is applied to his abdomen, and the belief that there are no countervailing facts with respect to his being in pain. As I suggested above, even in that circumstance the belief that Tom is in pain need not result from a chain of reasoning. Still, the belief that Tom winces when pressure is applied to his abdomen and the belief that there are no relevant countervailing facts may form part of the basis of your belief that Tom is in pain. For they may be implicated in, and, in the circumstances, necessary for, the causal sustenance of the latter. Any tendency on your part to cease to believe that Tom is in pain, induced, say, by your being told that he is not, would have to reckon with your belief that he winces under pressure to his abdomen. And should you come to think that the wincing could be explained without assuming Tom to be in pain, say by his having been tickled when pressure is applied to his abdomen, you would need some other reason to continue to believe that he is in pain, such as might be provided by a pained expression on his face. So even though the belief that Tom is in pain has not been generated from a chain of reasoning it could still derive its justification in part from the other beliefs mentioned in a way which mirrors abstract inferential links among the relevant contents. Indeed, even if the basis beliefs are involved in bringing it about that you believe that Tom is in pain rather than merely sustaining that belief, it does not follow that you must have inferred, in the sense of reasoned, that Tom is in pain from prior data. For the processes resulting in the formation of your belief that Tom is in pain may have taken place at a sub-personal level[20] without involving you in a chain of reasoning in any ordinary sense.

McDowell is struck, I think, by the phenomenological immediacy with which we could acquire the belief that Tom is in pain by looking at him. Hence the thought that inference conceived psychologically as involving a chain of reasoning need not be implicated. I am suggesting that though this thought is correct, patterns of inference, conceived abstractly along evidentialist lines, are still relevant even in the perceptual case. In the perceptual case some belief as to Tom's behaviour is involved and we cannot do justice to how it is involved unless we think of it as an element in the evidential basis of the belief that Tom is in pain.

There is another strand in McDowell's thinking in this area which I have not considered and which has to do with how to respond to scepticism. In this chapter as a whole I have deliberately steered clear of that topic, reserving it for fuller discussion in Chapter 7.

3.5. *Best Explanations*

My own approach to the current topic shares with the criterion theory the idea that the practice of applying the concept of pain presupposes various general evidential propositions linking pain behaviour with pain. I differ from criterion theorists in taking these propositions to be contingent, but I agree with such theorists in thinking that the legitimacy of believing them true does not derive from empirical support.

There is yet another approach to the topic according to which

[20] On the idea of sub-personal processes, see Dennett (1969), pp. 93 ff.

the general evidential propositions linking pain behaviour with pain are contingent and form part of folk psychology conceived as a theoretical framework in terms of which we explain and predict behaviour. Furthermore, according to this view, the justification for accepting the framework lies in the fact that it yields the best explanations available for human behaviour. Disenchantment with the criterion theory, and a general predilection for styles of explanation and of justification assumed to be characteristic of natural science, has led to this approach being extremely influential at the present time. I think it is radically mistaken, though a full treatment of the matter lies outwith the scope of this book.[21]

It is important to distinguish between the different elements of the approach, that is between the claim that folk psychology constitutes a theoretical explanatory framework and the claim that acceptance of the framework is justified because it provides the best explanations of behaviour. Even if folk psychology is in some sense a theoretical framework it is a further question whether we are justified in accepting it because of its explanatory power. In connection with this there is another important distinction between the framework itself and the particular explanations of behaviour which it yields. His being in pain may well be the best explanation for the fact that a person winces when pressure is applied to some region of his body. We have clear notions of what alternative explanations there might be, and it is relevant to our accepting that someone is in pain that we reject these alternatives. This much is accommodated by the account of 3.2. The important thing to note in the present context is that our notions of alternative explanations are built into the framework of folk psychology itself. They are not alternatives to the framework. They are among the explanations which the framework allows for. It is a different matter when we come to think of the framework as a whole. To say that the framework provides best ways of explaining behavioural phenomena, is to imply that it is better than competing alternatives,

[21] The general approach is mooted in Chihara and Fodor (1965) which is principally a critical discussion of criterion theories. See also Harman (1973), Paul Churchland (1979, 1984), and Stich (1983). Haldane (1988) is a critical treatment of the general approach focusing on Churchland and raising many questions which to my mind have not yet received adequate answers.

which in this case must mean alternatives to the framework. But we have no clear idea about what the competing alternatives might be. This is not to say that there could not be live alternatives to the prevailing framework. Some philosophers argue that a properly scientific understanding of the aetiology of behaviour is in the offing which will cast folk psychology aside. This is a highly speculative view venturing far beyond what we have a right to expect in the present state of understanding. But even supposing it should turn out that there are alternatives to folk psychology, that would not help to substantiate the claim that what justifies our accepting the framework is its being for now the best we have.

Justification is a causal notion. The proposed view when read with this in mind must be taken to imply that if we are justified in accepting folk psychology then we accept it at least in part because we believe that it is the best explanatory framework available. But this view is quite unrealistic from a psychological point of view. There is no evidence whatsoever that we adopt the framework for this reason. Indeed, it seems quite unrealistic to suppose that we accept folk psychology, as opposed to particular explanations which it yields, for any reason at all. There is in any case another way of viewing the matter which is more realistic from a psychological point of view. The folk-psychological framework includes psychological concepts as well as those general evidential propositions linking behaviour and the mental which I have suggested are normative for us. We do not think in terms of the framework because we have grounds for doing so. The framework itself determines what is a ground for the attributions of psychological states that we make in terms of the framework.

Views along these lines are apt to be regarded with suspicion on the grounds that they place what might be mere dogma or prejudice beyond the need for justification. I shall be taking up this matter at length in Chapter 6. Here I want to stress only that from the fact that we have no grounds, and no need of grounds, for thinking within the folk-psychological framework, it by no means follows that folk psychology is immune to radical revision. We saw earlier that evidential propositions which are normative for us now, and which we accept groundlessly, could conceivably be called into question. The same may be said for other normative propositions making up folk psychology. So the epistemological approach which I am commending should not be conceived as part of an attempt to show folk psychology to be immune to revision.

The view that our acceptance of the folk-psychological framework, as opposed to particular attributions of psychological states, is justified by the fact that it yields the best explanations of behaviour faces another difficulty. It does seem to presuppose that our cognitive predicament is one in which we can, in McDowell's words, suspend 'all attributions of psychological properties to others'. After all the view is meant to justify our thinking that others do have psychological states. The problem is that we conceive of the behaviour which folk psychology explains as essentially mind-involving even when not caused by the particular states we think it manifests. Folk psychology explains someone's going shopping, not his making such-and-such specific bodily movements. And even in the case of wincing, as we noted earlier, agreeing to this extent with McDowell, we think of the subject of wincing as a subject of psychological states. Behaviour conceived as being mind-involving can hardly provide us with useful evidence that people have minds.

4

Experience and Justification

4.1. *Some Problems*

There is a sense in which the theory of justification set out in Chapter 2 is regulative. Suppose that your belief that *p* derives its justification from your beliefs that *q, r,* . . . . In that case by the Rational Connection condition *JUS2'* *q, r,* . . . must constitute an unconditional reason for thinking that *p*. But, as we saw, it should be no mere fluke that this condition is satisfied. According to the Competence condition *JUS3* your basing your belief that *p* on your beliefs that *q, r,* . . . must be an exercise of competence on your part with respect to the patterns of inference which underwrite the fact that *q, r,* . . . constitute an unconditional reason for *p*. To have the required competence is a matter of being governed or, if you like, regulated by the relevant patterns of inference. The notion of being thus governed fills out the sense in which the theory of justification is regulative. Note that the idea is not that the theory itself regulates but rather that it builds in a condition of justified belief requiring you to be regulated by inference patterns which the inferential steps from *q, r,* . . . to *p* instantiate.

Not all theories of justification are regulative. There are reliability theories, for instance, which count beliefs as being justified if, roughly speaking, they are produced by processes which reliably yield true beliefs. On this view of the matter a subject may acquire a belief by such a process and thus satisfy the appropriate conditions of justification without in any sense having been guided by a requirement to form or maintain beliefs by reliable processes. Of course, a subject who has beliefs to the

[1] Much of this chapter derives from a paper, delivered to the Scots Philosophical Club meeting in Stirling in Dec. 1987, which is an early version of Millar (1989). I am grateful to those who were present then for discussion and encouragement.

effect that certain processes are reliable may adjust his or her thinking accordingly and thus be guided by these beliefs. But reliability theories do not in general require that beliefs are justified only if some belief as to the reliability of the process by which they were produced was appropriately in play. Indeed, such theories are usually presented as alternatives to regulative theories and to be preferable because they cope with cases of justified belief in which regulative constraints might be thought to have no role.[2]

An important class of such cases concerns what I shall call *E*-beliefs, that is to say, beliefs about the present environment which are at least partially based on current experience, such as the belief which you might have now that a book is in front of you. There are a number of problems here. A regulative theory might seem to require that when an *E*-belief derives its justification at least in part from current experience the subject must have regard to the experience. The idea would be that if there are regulative constraints on the sorts of experiences which can contribute to the justification of beliefs of a certain type then a subject can be guided by these constraints only if able to tell when current experience is of the right type for the given type of belief. This would require checking on current experience, but that is not something which in general we do when we have *E*-beliefs. When we reflect on cases in which beliefs derive justification from other beliefs this is hardly likely to seem a serious problem. In these cases the subject must indeed have some conception of what makes the basis beliefs appropriate. But there is no requirement to have the thought that the basis beliefs are appropriate. So there is no reason to expect that in the case where a belief derives its justification, at least in part, from current experience the subject should have a thought to the effect that the current experience is appropriate.

Other more serious problems arise for regulative theories in connection with particular views of experience. Some writers, most notably Quine, have thought that we can do all that needs to be done in cognitive psychology without positing experiences

[2] A non-regulative reliability theory is presented in some detail in Goldman (1986). Earlier discussions by Goldman on this topic include his (1976, 1979, 1985). The main inspiration for reliablity theories in recent years comes from Armstrong (1973). See also Swain (1981) and Nozick (1981).

as conscious occurrences.[3] All that we need are stimulations conceived as irradiations of nerve-endings standing in complex causal relations to beliefs. On this view conscious intermediaries between stimulations and beliefs have no explanatory, and thus no justificatory, role to play. It is difficult also on a regulative theory to accommodate the idea that stimulations have a justificatory role. Part of the problem is simply that we do not in fact evaluate *E*-beliefs in the light of the stimulations by which they are prompted. Indeed, we may competently form and evaluate *E*-beliefs while lacking any notion of what stimulations are. And there is another dimension to the problem posed by stimulations. A regulative theory can make sense of the idea that beliefs may derive their justification from other beliefs because it can make sense of there being a rational connection between the basis beliefs and the based belief. Such a connection obtains when the contents of the basis beliefs constitute an unconditional reason for thinking that the content of the based belief is true. It is not clear how, lacking propositional contents, stimulations could have a justificatory role in relation to beliefs.

This last problem would also arise if experiences are conceived as sensations and sensations are contrasted with propositional attitudes. Thus Donald Davidson writes[4],

> The relation between a sensation and a belief cannot be logical, since sensations are not beliefs or other propositional attitudes. What then is the relation? The answer is, I think, obvious: the relation is causal. Sensations cause some beliefs and in *this* sense are the basis or ground of those beliefs. But a causal explanation of belief does not show how or why the belief is justified.[5]

Reading the phrase 'logical relation' liberally as capturing the sense of my 'rational connection', Davidson's point could be developed in terms of the general approach to derivative justification set out in Chapter 2. It is tempting to generalize that approach so that it yields the following view: If a belief derives its justification at least in part from mental state *S*, then at the very least something analogous to the Basing, Rational Connection, and Competence conditions must be satisfied. Otherwise,

[3] See e.g. Quine (1960, 1973, 1975).
[4] Davidson (1983), repr. in LePore (1986). Page references are to the latter edn.
[5] Davidson (1983), p. 311.

it is difficult to see how *S* could have a justificatory rather than merely a causal role. But then it would seem that mental states having a justificatory role should be propositional attitudes. As yet we have no clear idea of how states other than propositional attitudes could satisfy either the Rational Connection or Competence conditions. If Davidson is right sensations would not fit the bill.

One way of responding to what I shall call *Davidson's problem*[6] would be to criticize the underlying assumption that the class of sensations and the class of propositional attitudes are mutually exclusive. Experiences could be treated as hybrids which have both sensational and propositional dimensions. The differences between experiences and itches and experiences and beliefs can readily be accommodated within such a view. Itches could be regarded as pure sensations and beliefs, if they have no distinctive phenomenology, as pure propositional attitudes. Defenders of the view that experiences have a justificatory role could avail themselves of this approach though there would still remain the task of spelling out the nature of the rational connections which may hold between experiences and beliefs and making it plausible that we have the required kind of competence.

This approach is not open to me since I have argued at some length in Chapter 1 that experiences are not properly conceived as propositional attitudes. None the less, I contend that we may plausibly account for how experiences could have a justificatory role rather than merely a causal role. The central idea is that there are analogues of the Rational Connection and Competence conditions which apply to *E*-beliefs. The discussions of previous chapters bear directly on the concerns of this chapter in that, among other things, they challenge us to to show how Davidson's problem can be met using the conception of sensory experience presented in Chapter 1 while keeping to the spirit of the account of justified belief developed in Chapters 2 and 3. Before getting down to details I shall argue that we do have reason to think of experiences as contributing to the justification of beliefs.

[6] I focus on Davidson because he succinctly expresses the thought that if experiences are not propositional attitudes they cannot contribute to justification. Others have discussed the problem of whether experiences can have a justificatory role. See e.g. Watkins (1984), ch. 7, and Pollock (1987).

4.2. *Why think that Experiences contribute to the Justification of Beliefs?*

If experiences contribute to the justification of *E*-beliefs then we should be able to make sense of the idea that beliefs can be legitimately or illegitimately based on current experience or on current experience in a context of currently held beliefs. That is to say, in addition to evaluating *E*-beliefs with respect to truth and falsity, we must be able to evaluate them with respect to justification where this latter type of evaluation takes into account the current experiences on which the *E*-beliefs are in part based. Moreover, if experiences contribute to the justification of beliefs in a regulative way, then the subjects of *E*-beliefs must be capable of appraising these beliefs in the light of the relevant experiences.

Suppose that Bill, who is short-sighted, is standing at a bus stop. Looking into the distance he comes to believe that a number 3 bus is on its way. It may be true that such a bus is coming, but if it is far enough away you may think that Bill was not in a position to judge that this is so by sight. The thought would be that if he was relying on sight Bill was not justified in believing that a number 3 bus was coming. It might be suggested that the reason that Bill was not in a position to tell that a number 3 was coming is simply that his perceptual mechanism is not reliable over distances of a certain length. It need not be denied that experiences occur in perception. The point is that such experiences as one may be said to possess need not be conceived as having a regulative justificatory role in relation to beliefs. The crucial consideration, according to this line of thought, is the reliability of the relevant perceptual mechanism, in this case sight.

The trouble with this way of conceiving the matter is that it does not take into account a kind of evaluation of his belief that Bill himself can subsequently make. Suppose that, having come to think that a number 3 is coming, Bill's attention is distracted by someone with whom he enters into conversation. The bus comes and goes and Bill's companion asks which bus it was. Bill begins to wonder whether it was really a number 3. Clearly, he might be led to such a doubt by consideration of his short-sightedness and the distance involved. But equally clearly his doubt might have its source in his recollection of the visual experience he had as he looked at the bus. He may not even realize that he is short-sighted but he can, as it were, replay in imagination the experience he had and come to realize that he did not clearly discern the numeral on the bus. As William Lyons has observed,[7] such replay is not to be understood as the calling up of an image which may then be inspected with the inner eye, whatever that might be. It is the production in imagination of something which is akin to the original experience. But it is not an object of perception any more than the original experience was. Visual replay of this kind could be the basis of Bill's doubt that the approaching bus was a number 3. But now, a doubt of this kind is not just a doubt as to the truth of what he formerly believed. It is a doubt as to the truth of the belief deriving from a doubt as to whether his experience was such as to put him in a position to believe that a number 3 was approaching. We may coherently suppose the latter doubt to remain even if it were settled on other grounds that the belief was true.

The example serves to highlight the fact that we can readily make sense of the idea that your current experience may be relevant to whether a belief based on that experience is justified. But it also brings out the fact that a subject can evaluate his own beliefs in the light of the experiences which prompted them. This is important for our project for unless it were so it could hardly be plausible to suppose that the formation and maintenance of beliefs can be guided by considerations relating to the appropriateness of the experiences on which they were at least initially based.

This line of thought may be developed further drawing on distinctions made in Chapter 1. The key distinctions were these:

> An experience is such that *it seems to the subject that an F is there* if and only if it is such that in the absence of countervailing considerations the subject would believe that an *F* is there.
>
> An experience in the modality of *M* is *F-type* if and only if it satisfies the following condition: it is of a type such that in suitable environmental conditions an *F* would produce an

[7] See Lyons (1986) for an extensive discussion of 'replay'.

experience of that type in an observer who is suitably positioned and orientated and whose sense of *M* is normal (in short, if and only if it is of the type that *F*s yield).

An experience is *of an F* if and only if it is *F*-type and such that it seems to the subject that an *F* is there.

Let us focus for the moment on what it is to recall a past experience, considering in particular what account we should give of Bill's visually recalling the experience he had as he looked at the bus in the distance. Suppose we could only avail ourselves of the notion that the experience Bill had as he looked at the bus was such that it seemed to him that a number 3 bus was coming. In that case his subsequent recollection could only be a matter of recalling having had an experience such that it seemed that a number 3 bus was coming. But if the experience were recalled only *qua* bearer of the content that a number 3 bus is coming then there would be nothing about the recollection which could account for Bill's doubting on its basis that he was in a position to believe the content true. To account for Bill's subsequent evaluation we must suppose that, prompted by the replay of his past experience, he comes to realize that he did not clearly discern the numeral on the bus and so was not in a position to believe on the basis of his experience that a number 3 was coming. This realization is only possible because Bill has a conception of what the experience would have had to be like to put him in a position to believe as he did. This conception, however, is not the conception of an experience which is such that it seems to the subject that a number 3 bus is coming, it is rather a conception of the experience's being of a certain phenomenal type, the type which approaching number 3 buses yield when the numeral on the front is clearly discernible.

In 1.5 I suggested that we should think of experiences as interacting with conceptual capacities in, roughly speaking, the following way: Let us say that the concept of an *F* is *experiential* if it is such that its mastery enables one to tell from the appearance of a thing whether or not it is an instance. Suppose that the concept of an *F* is experiential. The idea is that for subjects who possess the concept, *F*-type experiences are apt to be such that it seems to the subject that an *F* is there, where the explanation for this lies in those capacities which are constitutive of the concept's mastery. In the example just considered we have a case in which the content of an experience and its phenomenal type are out of kilter. The natural explanation for this is that the relevant concept is misapplied. Bill applies the concept of an approaching number 3 bus to the present scene. The trouble is that he does so in response to an experience of the wrong type. The underlying idea is that experiences may take on the content that an *F* is there through the exercise of the conceptual capacities in which mastery of the relevant concept consists. As we saw previously, *F*-type experiences may fail to be such that it seems to the subject that an *F* is there, either because the subject lacks the concept of an *F* or because the experience, for some reason or another, does not engage with the corresponding conceptual capacities. Now we see that the capacities corresponding to the concept of an *F* may be engaged by an experience of the wrong type, in particular by an experience which is not *F*-type. Given the fallibility of our capacities these different ways in which phenomenal type and content can fail to mesh should come as no surprise.

Another example provides further illustration of the faulty exercise of a conceptual capacity in response to an experience of the wrong type. Nectarines look a bit like red apples. Even so, nectarines and apples are visually distinguishable if looked at carefully. We can make sense of the idea that an experience is (red apples)-type but not nectarines-type, and vice versa. Now, you can be in a situation in which you believe you are looking at red apples when in fact you are looking at nectarines. This conceivably could happen if on looking at the nectarines you received an experience which was (red apples)-type but not nectarines-type. That would be a rather exotic case suggestive of some defect in your perceptual mechanism. In the kind of case I have in mind you have an experience such that it seems to you that red apples are before you, although in fact there are nectarines, and the fault lies with your beliefs rather than in your senses. Two cases are distinguishable. The first is where you take in the fruits in a quick passing glance, perhaps in some location where you habitually expect red apples. Given a not unreasonably strict reading of the suitability conditions associated with the typology we are using, the experience may be neither (red apples)-type nor nectarines-type, and yet it may be such as to lead you to believe that apples are there. The second case is where you do have a nectarines-type experience but your attention is distracted by conversation and you are not concentrating on what you are looking at. You may be focusing on the fruits all right but you are not attending *in thought* to what you see. Whereas in this case you do see properly what you are looking at, in the first case you do not. In both cases, you are too quick to believe that apples are there. The experience is such that it seems that red apples are before you and, there being no countervailing facts, so far as you know, that is what you believe. But the experience is not of a type which is apt for the proper engagement of the relevant conceptual capacities.

These considerations show that we have a grasp of the phenomenal types of our experiences and of their aptness for bearing certain propositional contents. But they also provide us with the beginnings of a defence of the view that experiences can have a genuinely justificatory role. Experiences do cause us to have beliefs but they do so by interacting with conceptual capacities. The formation or maintenance of beliefs whose justification derives in part from current experience must result from the competent exercise of these capacities.

4.3. *How Experiences can have a Justificatory Role*

In the case where a belief derives its justification from other beliefs the Rational Connection condition must be satisfied: the contents of the basis beliefs must constitute an unconditional reason for the content of the based belief. Also, the Competence condition must be satisfied: In basing the belief in question in the way he does the subject must be exercising conceptual capacities relating to the relevant concepts, and that means exercising inferential competence with respect to the relevant inference patterns. As we saw in 4.1 Davidson's problem turns on the thought that experiences, conceived as lacking intrinsic propositional contents, do not have rational as opposed to merely causal connections with beliefs. The previous discussion has already given us reason to resist this thought via the idea that experience types may or may not be appropriate for the beliefs which are in part based upon them. In this section I develop the argument further, arguing that we should countenance quasi-inferential links between experience types and belief contents, as well as conceptual capacities informed by a tacit appreciation of these links. This will enable us to formulate the analogues of the Rational Connection and Competence conditions which we are seeking.

Up to this point I have taken a liberal view of the sorts of concepts which can be experiential in the sense that their mastery enables the subject to tell that something is an instance from its appearance. Thus I have been happy to treat concepts of familiar natural kinds as being experiential as well as colour concepts like that of something red. I shall explore this matter at length in the next two sections. For the present I want to focus on what I shall call *concepts of appearances*. Examples would be the concepts of a thing having the look of an apple, the feel of a peach, the sound of rushing water, and so forth. It is surely unproblematic that we can tell from the visual appearance of something that it at least has the look of an apple. I shall examine how beliefs to the effect that something has the look of an *F* may derive their justification, at least in part, from current experience.[8]

Let us first of all think of how you might actually form a belief about the look of something before you in response to current experience. Suppose that you have a (thing having the look of a red apple)-type visual experience. Since this type of experience is by our conventions just the type which red apples yield, though they may be produced by things which are not red apples, we may describe the experience in question simply as (red apples)-type. Given that you have such an experience under what conditions would you believe that something having the look of a red apple is there? The answer suggested by the discussion thus far is this: If you have the concept of something having the look of a red apple and you are not subject to distractions, that is, influences which might as in the nectarines case lead you to mistaken judgements, then it will

[8] In 1.6 I used the phrase 'look of an *F*' in such a way that one could possess the concept of the look of an *F* without possessing the concept of an *F*. Here I return to more familiar usage. I take it that the property we ascribe to something when we say it has the look of an *F* is simply the property of having various visible characteristics. In describing these characteristics as the look of an *F* we simply think of them as characteristics possessed by *F*s.

seem to you that something having the look of a red apple is there. You will, therefore, believe that such a thing is there in the absence of countervailing considerations. We need to take a closer look at what is meant by saying that countervailing considerations are absent.

Clearly you would not believe that something having the look of a red apple is there if you had beliefs to the effect that certain countervailing facts obtain. These would be facts which either explain your having a (red apple)-type experience without assuming that a thing which has the look of a red apple is there, or which independently cast doubt on whether such a thing is there. It might be suggested then that all that is required for you to believe that something having the look of a red apple is there is that you lack a belief that countervailing facts obtain. But there is an important difference between merely lacking such a belief and having at some level taken into account whether countervailing facts obtain. Assuming that you have a mastery of the concept in question you will be aware of a range of possibilities in which countervailing facts obtain and you will be, as it were, geared up to withholding belief in circumstances where such facts might well obtain. For instance, in old-fashioned shops where the interior lighting distorts the colours of things you may think twice about whether it is indeed something having the look of a red apple which you see. (The issue, remember, is not whether something which has the look of a red apple is a red apple but whether something before you has the look of a red apple.) So if you lack a belief that countervailing facts obtain on some occasion when you have the experience under consideration it will not be because you do not know what would count as countervailing or are indifferent to such matters but rather because one of two alternatives obtains. The first is that no countervailing facts come to your attention. Even then you will be primed to take up the default position of taking it for granted, albeit tacitly, that no countervailing facts obtain. The other alternative is that something makes you suspect that countervailing facts obtain. You would then check out the situation to satisfy yourself that none does. The upshot is that we may clarify the notion of its seeming to you that something having the look of a red apple is there. This is to be taken as meaning that you would believe that something having the look of a red apple is there so long as you believe that there are no relevant countervailing facts.

Note that it is quite natural to think of you as believing that no countervailing facts obtain even though the issue of whether they do has not occurred to you. What supports the claim that you do so believe is that you are disposed to deny that countervailing facts obtain if the question is put and the best explanation of your being so disposed, in the circumstances in question, is that you actually believe that there are no such facts. It seems possible that a person should be disposed to deny that *p* if the question were put, yet not already believe not-*p*. For instance, you may be disposed to deny that you are a two-headed dragon from the planet Zog, if the question were put, yet we would have some hesitation, I think, in ascribing to you on that basis a belief that you are not a two-headed dragon from the planet Zog prior to any denial you might make. Your preparedness to make the denial is adequately explained in terms of a general preparedness unhesitatingly to deny obvious falsehoods. But the case in hand is one in which (i) there is something at stake, namely whether something having the look of a red apple is before you, (ii) there being such-and-such facts would create a doubt that there is such a thing before you, and (iii) you appreciate that (ii) is true. In these circumstances it seems natural to think of you as taking for granted, and thus believing, that there are no relevant countervailing facts even if you give the matter no thought. The underlying idea is that given (iii), and barring some cognitive impairment, it would be difficult to account for your believing that something having the look of a red apple is before you were it not assumed that you take for granted that there are no relevant countervailing facts.[9]

Bearing these points in mind we can represent by means of a diagram a transition of the sort described in the example from the occurrence of an experience to the formation of a belief about what is before you in response to that experience (Figure 1). Our example is of a case in which a belief is brought about by a current experience but the diagram may be taken to cover cases in which a belief is sustained by current experience. We are interested in the conditions under which a belief formed in this

[9] Related perplexities concerning belief are explored in Lycan (1986).

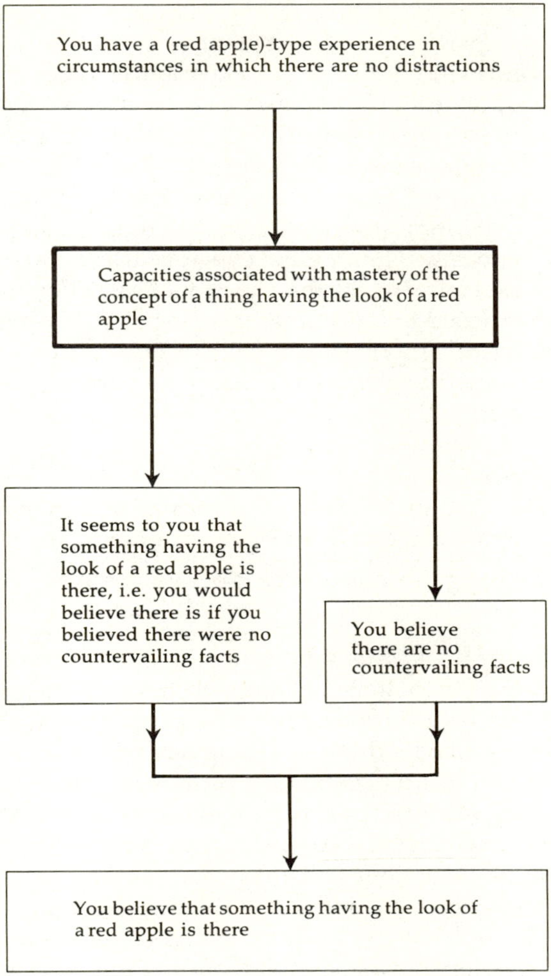

FIG. 1

way would be justified. In the example the input experience was surely appropriate for the belief which was formed in response to it. As we have seen, input experiences may be inappropriate for the beliefs based upon them. Recall the examples of Bill at the bus-stop and of the nectarines mistaken for apples. The possibility of correct or incorrect applications of concepts in response to experience makes it natural to conceive of there being inference-like links from experience types to belief contents. I shall call these links *quasi-inferences*. Some preliminaries will help to characterize the kind of quasi-inferential link relating to our last example. As in 1.7 I use '$T(F)$' to denote the type to which F-type experiences belong. The relevant modality may be indicated with a prefix, thus 'Visual $T(F)$'. A subject may conceive of an F-type experience as being his own. In that case he conceives of the experience as belonging to the type $T(F)$ as indexed to himself, that is, as belonging to the type $T(F)_{\text{self}}$. Quasi-inferences whose conclusions are to the effect that there is something before one having a particular look take the following general form.

Q Visual $T(F)_{\text{self}}$

There are no countervailing facts with respect to there being a thing having the look of an F before oneself

---

A thing having the look of an F is before oneself.

It is important to read this schema in the light of the previous discussion. *Q* is a pattern relating abstract entities, namely experience types and propositions. The proposal is that part of what makes your belief that something having the look of a red apple before you justified is that the proposition that something having the look of a red apple before you is quasi-inferable from the type of your current experience and the proposition that there are no relevant countervailing facts. In other words, the quasi-inference which the formation of your belief mirrors is an instance of *Q*. By analogy with the inference patterns we have considered previously we may think of the experience type and the proposition relating to countervailing facts as comprising a special kind of unconditional yet inconclusive reason for the corresponding conclusion—what could be called an experiential reason. This is made natural by the fact that a person who has an F-type experience and who legitimately takes it for granted that there are no relevant countervailing facts may be said to have an unconditional reason to believe that a thing having the look of an F is there. Note also that *Q* is truth-conducive in a sense closely analogous to that introduced in 2.4. That is to say, quasi-inferences in the psychological sense—transitions from an experience and belief to a belief—instantiating *Q* and having a true input belief would more often than not yield true output beliefs.

Note that *Q* relates to the formation and maintenance of a subject's beliefs on the basis of that subject's current experience. Although it may govern many people, what the pattern requires of a subject concerns that subject's experience and the beliefs which that subject bases on that experience.

There arises now the question of how *Q* relates to particular concepts which may be applied in response to current experience. The natural suggestion is surely that *Q* is an introduction pattern which partially characterizes the inferential role of the concept of the look of something. Thus if you possess that concept you must be governed by *Q*. This means that you must manage your beliefs and evaluate beliefs generally in ways which respect quasi-inferences instantiating *Q*. A great deal more needs to be said about the relation between concepts and quasi-inferences, but already we are in a position to formulate a number of conditions which need to be satisfied if *A*'s belief that an *F* is there is justified and derives its justification from a current experience *e* and a belief to the effect that there are no relevant countervailing facts.

First, we have a Basing condition demanding that *A* believe that an *F* is there because he has *e* and believes that there are no countervailing facts. Secondly, we have a Rational Connection condition demanding that there be an appropriate quasi-inferential link between the proposition that an *F* is there, the type of *e*, and the proposition that there are no relevant countervailing facts. This requirement would be satisfied if the experience is *F*-type. Thirdly, we have a Competence condition. *A*'s believing that an *F* is there on the basis of *e* and his belief that there are no countervailing facts must be the outcome of the exercise of competence on his part in employing the concept of an *F*. Fourthly, we have a Basis condition. *A* must be in a position to take it for granted that there are no countervailing facts with respect to there being an *F* before him. He may have taken steps to satisfy himself that this is so but the account does not require him to have done so. As I suggested above a person may take up the default position of taking it for granted that there are no countervailing facts in circumstances in which nothing occurs which suggests that such facts might obtain. Any account of justification which is to be psychologically realistic and reflect our ordinary evaluative practice must allow that this is legitimate and suffices to meet the Basis condition. We do not require a separate clause in the Basis condition to deal with the token experience *e*. That is because there can be no question of whether you ought to have *e* in the way that there can be a question of whether you ought to believe that there are countervailing facts. Recall, however, that the Rational Connection condition requires that *e* be of an appropriate type.

These conditions are in obvious ways analogous to our conditions for the case in which a belief derives its justification from other beliefs. They give content to the claim that experiences not merely cause beliefs but contribute to their justification, and thus show how the challenge posed by Davidson's problem can be met while keeping to the spirit of the general approach to justification with which we started.

Do we really need the notion of a quasi-inference to account for the justification of *E*-beliefs? An alternative proposal would be that all we need are straightforward inferences from propositions about experience to propositions about what is before the subject. We already have to hand an account of inference from evidence which may seem to fit the bill nicely. In Chapters 2 and 3 I discussed inferences instantiating the following pattern.

> *e*
>
> *e* is strong fallible evidence for *h*.
>
> There are no relevant countervailing facts with respect to *h*.
>
> ———————————————————————————
>
> *h*

The alternative proposal has it that we can account for the justification of *E*-beliefs in terms of inferences instantiating the above pattern and having the following more specific form.

E *A* has an *F*-type experience.

A's having an *F*-type experience is strong fallible evidence that something having the look of an *F* is before *A*.

There are no relevant countervailing facts with respect to there being something having the look of an *F* before *A*.

Something having the look of an *F* is before *A*.

My own view of the matter is that while we do recognize the legitimacy of inferences of this sort we still need quasi-inferences to account for the justification of *E*-beliefs. An important consideration here is that *E* relates to cases in which beliefs about what is before one are based on beliefs as to the type of a subject's experience together with auxiliary beliefs concerning an evidential link and associated countervailing facts. One obvious problem is that it is far from clear that ordinary *E*-beliefs are based on beliefs as to the type of one's own current experience. Indeed, it is not even clear that we have such beliefs in ordinary situations in which we form beliefs in response to current experience. Another problem is that the alternative proposal would require some account of the legitimacy of these problematic beliefs. The question would then be whether this could plausibly be done without positing something like quasi-inferences. But aside from these considerations the fact remains that the transitions we make from experiences to beliefs about what is before us do seem to be evaluable with respect to justification. When Bill at the bus-stop reflects on the experience he had on looking at the approaching bus, he forms a belief as to its type, but what he is evaluating is whether the past experience, as opposed to a belief he had about that experience at the time he had it, put him in a position legitimately to believe that a number 3 was approaching. It is that kind of evaluation which is naturally explained in terms of quasi-inferences and not explained in terms of inferences instantiating *E*.

Having said all that it remains true that we do sometimes go through chains of reasoning which have regard to *E*. If what you seem to be looking at is very odd it becomes for you a live question whether you should take your experience at face value. Imagine, for instance, being in a wood at night and seeming to see a strange creature having the look of a leprechaun. Suppose this creature has an appearance which is so extraordinary as to make it at least doubtful that you should trust your senses. Realizing this you think to yourself that the experience you have is just as it would be if there were something having the look of a leprechaun before you. In other words, you think to yourself that your current visual experience is leprechaun-type. Then you reason that it would be very odd to have such an experience if there were not something having the look of a leprechaun before you, a thought to the effect that the occurrence of such an experience is strong fallible evidence for the presence of such a creature. But being a cautious person you look at other possibilities. You wonder if you have been working too hard lately, beginning to crack up, and so forth, but you decide that things are not that bad. You wonder if the light is playing tricks with you and decide that it is not. After further reflections in this vein you conclude, as you might say, that there is no reason to doubt your senses, which is tantamount to concluding that there are no relevant countervailing facts. So, finally, you conclude that after all there is before you something having the look of a leprechaun.

There is no difficulty then in the idea that we are governed by the inference pattern *E*. In ordinary cases of *E*-belief we do not, of course, reason in the way just illustrated. Nevertheless, *E* does have a bearing on the ordinary case.

Something is missing from the account given so far. We need to consider yet again the notion of countervailing facts. What makes the fact that the lighting conditions are peculiar relevant to whether there are countervailing facts with respect to the hypothesis that something before you has the look of a red apple? Part of the answer is, obviously, that such conditions might explain your having a (red apple)-type experience without assuming that an object of the relevant sort is present. If this were in fact the explanation for your having the experience in question then the presumption that something having the look of a red apple is before you would be undermined. But that presumption is created because the occurrence of a (red apple)-type experience is strong fallible evidence that something having the look of a red apple is present. So the notion of countervailing facts with respect to a hypothesis, in this context as elsewhere, operates in tandem with a concept dealing with evidence for that hypothesis. If you possess a concept of countervailing facts with respect to *h* you must possess an associated concept of strong fallible evidence for *h*. I argued in Chapter 2 that these tandem concepts are exhibited by a general inference pattern which relates strong fallible evidence with a hypothesis. We have just seen that *E* is a special case. The conclusion to be drawn is that if you possess the concept of countervailing facts relevant in cases covered by *E* then you must be governed by *E*.

Let us think again about a case in which you form a belief that something having the look of an *F* is before you, unreflectively, in response to a current *F*-type experience. Our account has it that you must believe that there are no relevant countervailing facts. These are to be conceived as facts which undermine the presumption that an *F* is before you. Thus anything which would explain your having a *F*-type experience, even if no *F* is there, would be countervailing. In view of this it might seem that you must believe that your current experience is *F*-type, but this is more than the account requires. You must, indeed, take it for granted that your current experience is of a type the occurrence of which creates a presumption that an *F* is before you. But you may do so not because you have formed a belief that the experience is *F*-type or any other specific type, but rather because you have a standing belief that in circumstances such as this, if you have taken due care, have not been distracted, and so forth, your experience will be appropriate for the beliefs which it disposes you to have.

If I am right in thinking it doubtful that we routinely form beliefs as to the type of our current experience then it could well be a virtue of the account I have given of the justification of *E*-beliefs that it does not require us to have such beliefs. On the other hand, we should avoid the extreme of supposing that there is something especially problematic about forming beliefs concerning the types of our experiences. My account requires that we do form such beliefs when we evaluate *E*-beliefs in the light of the experiences which prompted them. A source of unease about these beliefs may be the assumption that to have them would require the employment of sophisticated categories which could not be imputed to ordinary subjects. But if the beliefs in question have to do with types of experiences according to the *F*-type typology there would seem to be no problem. So far as (red thing)-type experiences are concerned the subject needs the concept of a red thing and a concept of the sorts of experiences that red things yield. There is no need of concepts of sensational properties whether as conceived in 1.7 or in any other way.[10]

4.4. *Experiential Concepts*

In the last section I argued that concepts of appearances are exhibited by quasi-inferential patterns. In this section I shall consider more generally the relation between concepts and quasi-inference patterns. This will serve to tie up loose ends and also to explore some interesting issues relating to natural-kind concepts and colour concepts.

If you are justified in believing that something having the look of an *F* is before you in the manner considered in the last section then I shall say that the belief in question is *Q*-justified. You can, for instance, be *Q*-justified in believing that something having the look of an apple is before you. It does not follow that you can be *Q*-justified in believing that an apple is before you. It is true that we think of apples as having a fairly distinctive visual appearance. That is to say, we believe that most things which have the look of an apple are apples. So we take it for granted, no doubt legitimately, that a thing's having the look of an apple is strong fallible evidence that it is an apple. And as with other cases of inference from strong fallible evidence we need to reckon in the standard way with the possibility of there being countervailing facts.

It is clearly contingent that the typical visual appearance of apples is fairly distinctive of apples. Realistic visually apple-like non-apples are rare, but if it should come about that there are at least as many fool's apples as there are apples it would no longer be true that the visual appearance of apples is fairly distinctive. If we discovered this to be so we would no longer judge that a

[10] Pollock points out that when we walk into a room we do not think things like 'A bright red trapezoidal shape appears in the right hand corner of my visual field' (Pollock (1987), p. 62). The remark is germane in the context of Pollock's discussion of foundationalism. But it does not show that we do not from time to time make use of concepts of types of experience as these are conceived in this section.

thing is an apple just from its visual appearance, yet there is no reason to suppose that in that event our concept of an apple would have changed. A person who possesses the concept is not bound to believe that the familiar visual appearance we associate with instances is fairly distinctive.

In the respect just mentioned the concept of an apple is akin to the concept of pain. I argued in 3.2 that although it is built into the concept of pain that pains are apt to cause certain behaviours it is not built into the concept that these behaviours are usually caused by pain. Although it happens to be true that the familiar pain behaviours are usually caused by pain, it could come about, and we could discover, that this is no longer true of say, wincing. In that event, it would no longer be possible to tell that someone is in pain just from their wincing. As things are we have a mode of applying the concept which presupposes that wincing is strong fallible evidence of pain. If we were to discover that presupposition to be false, or discover that it has become false, then the relevant mode of applying the concept would have to change, though the concept could remain the same. This is what motivated the distinction made earlier between possessing a concept and employing some particular mode of application of the concept (3.2). Similar points hold for the concept of an apple. We have a mode of applying the concept which presupposes that a thing's having the look of an apple is strong fallible evidence that it is an apple. But in a world with as many fool's apples as apples this evidential link would not obtain.

To have a mastery of the concept of an apple in what I called the broad sense (3.2) you must have those capacities which go with possessing the concept plus the ability to employ the concept in line with prevailing modes of application, including that just considered, which those who possess the concept are not necessarily committed to recognizing as legitimate. This enables us to do justice to two intuitions which prima facie are in conflict. The first is that a mastery of the concept of an apple involves the ability to tell that something is an apple from its visual appearance. The other is that one may possess the concept of an apple and thus have a mastery of it, yet not be able to tell that things are apples from their visual appearance. To do justice to the first intuition we need the notion of broad mastery in the sense explained. To do justice to the second, we need the notion of narrow mastery, that is, the mastery which defines what it is merely to possess a concept.

Turning now to colour concepts it seems to be built into the concept of something red that red things have a distinctive visual appearance. A thing which is red has the look of a red thing and a thing which has the look of a red thing is red. In fact the inferential role of the concept is characterized in part by the inference patterns

X is red	*X* has the look of a red thing
X has the look of a red thing	*X* is red

This reflects the fact that to believe that something has the look of something red is just to believe that it is red. So if you are *Q*-justified in believing that something before you has the look of a red thing you are *Q*-justified in believing it is red. It needs to be borne in mind that to have the look of something red is to yield (red thing)-type experiences, where that means to produce such experiences in the usual normality and suitability conditions. There is also a sense in which a thing can look red and not be red, but in that sense to look red is a matter of producing (red thing)-type experiences though not necessarily in the usual normality and suitability conditions.

It might be suggested that one could possess the concept of something red yet not possess the concept of something which looks red. But here again it is important to note that to look red is to yield (red thing)-type visual experiences. These are just the sorts of experiences which someone who has the concept of something red must know to be appropriate for *Q*-justified beliefs that something red is present. Lacking such knowledge one would not be able to evaluate such beliefs, yet that ability is partially constitutive of what it is to possess the concept of something red. So there is no possessing the concept of something red without a notion of the sorts of experiences which red things yield, that is, of the way red things look.

Both the concept of an apple and the concept of something red are experiential in the sense explained in 4.2, which is to say that the mastery of these concepts enables one to tell that something is an instance from its appearance. But the concept of something red is *strongly experiential* in that narrow mastery suffices to tell that something is an instance from its visual appearance. A corollary of this is that beliefs to the effect that an instance is present can be *Q*-justified. The concept of an apple, on the other hand, is *weakly experiential*. Broad mastery incorporating our actual modes of applying the concept does enable one to tell that something is an instance from its appearance. Thus beliefs to the effect that something before one is an apple can be justified in a manner which essentially involves a *Q*-justified belief that the thing in question has the look of an apple. But the concept of an apple is *only* weakly experiential. Narrow mastery does not suffice to enable one to tell that something is an instance from its appearance.

We noted in the last section that if you are governed by the quasi-inference pattern *Q* then you need to possess concepts of relevant countervailing facts. If you have a concept of countervailing facts with respect to the presumption that an *F* is before you which would be created by your having an *F*-type experience, then you are committed to thinking of the occurrence of *F*-type experiences as strong fallible evidence that an *F* is there. What is the status of such evidential propositions in cases where the concept of an *F* is strongly experiential? Let us focus again on the concept of something red. Is it contingent that the occurrence of (red thing)-type experiences is strong fallible evidence of the presence of something red? In support of an affirmative answer we might try the following argument. Imagine that whenever we encounter a thing which we would actually call red the optical properties of the intervening medium are subject to localized alien-induced distortion. The things encountered are not red, because under the right suitability and normality conditions they would not produce (red thing)-type experiences. Yet the resulting experiences are still (red thing)-type, for they are the type which red things would yield, that is, would produce in the right suitability and normality conditions. So even though red things necessarily have a distinctive visual appearance, the look of red things, nevertheless it could be that the occurrence of (red thing)-type experiences is not strong fallible evidence of the presence of red things. The point is not that there can be fool's red things, just as there can be fool's apples. That is ruled out by the fact that the concept of a red thing is the concept of something having the look of a red thing. The point is rather that there can be things which produce (red thing)-type experiences but which are not red. This view retains the connection noted above between the look of a thing and the visual experiences which it yields. Red things are things which yield (red thing)-type experiences, that is, under the right suitability and normality conditions they would produce such experiences. It is just that a thing which is not red can also produce such experiences in conditions which are not of that sort.

This argument has a certain charm, but I am persuaded that it is unsound. We are to think of the condition which is supposed to result in non-red things producing (red thing)-type experiences as an interference. That is crucial to the argument, since it has to lend substance to the claim that the supposedly unreliable (red thing)-type experiences are produced in conditions which do not reveal the true appearance of the things which produce them. The problem is that we lose a grip on the idea that the condition in question is an interference when it has a stable and widespread role in the production of (red thing)-type experiences. We could be misled into thinking that we have a clear idea of how the condition could be interference by the fact that in the world as we conceive it to be there is nothing peculiar about the media through which light is reflected from the things we call red. But that does not suffice to sustain the notion that in a world in which the condition had the stable and widespread role it would be interference. Redness is a dispositional property of objects in a set-up which includes the surrounding medium and perceivers. In the imagined world the 'interfering' condition is a stable feature of the set-up. There is no reason to exclude it from the right suitability conditions and no reason for denying that (red thing)-type experiences in such a world are reliably indicative of the presence of red things.[11]

I conclude that it is not merely contingent but necessary that

[11] Wright (1988) explores closely related issues. See his discussion of the idea that the extension of the term 'red' is determined by our responses to certain things in appropriate conditions. See also the remarks in McGinn (1983), pp. 12 ff., to the effect that objects may look red in virtue of different categorical bases.

the occurrence of (red thing)-type experiences is strong fallible evidence of the presence of red things. Moreover, anyone who possesses the concept of something red is committed to holding that this evidential link obtains. This reflects the fact that it is partially constitutive of being red that red things yield experiences of a type the occurrence of which is strong fallible evidence of the presence of something red. Analogous points hold for all strongly experiential concepts. Thus necessarily the occurrence of blackcurrant-type gustatory experiences is strong fallible evidence of the presence of things having the taste of blackcurrants.

In 1.4 I argued that if you know what something looks like (what look it has) you must know what types of visual experiences it yields. I stressed that the knowledge required is not just a matter of having enjoyed experiences of the type in question. It requires you to know that they are of the type which such things yield. The argument to this effect turned crucially on the assumption that *E*-beliefs to the effect that a thing has the look of, say, a thrush, are subject to appraisal with respect to justification in the light of the experiences on which they are in part based. To now how thrushes look essentially involves the ability to make such appraisals and therefore requires a grasp of the types of experiences which thrushes yield. In the light of the discussion in this chapter of the justification of *E*-beliefs, this should seem less mysterious than it may have done at that early stage of the enquiry. We now have an account of how the experiences which things of a certain type yield can figure in the derived justification of an *E*-belief that a thing of the type is present.

4.5. *More on Natural Kinds*

I argued in the last section that the concept of an apple is only weakly experiential. It remains an open possibility that possession of the concept incurs a commitment to holding that if a thing is an apple then it is a member of a class of fruits which typically have the familiar visual appearance. Even if the familiar visual appearance is not fairly distinctive, in that most things which have it are apples, it might still be true and indeed necessarily true that apples typically have it.

There is a view of natural-kind concepts made familiar by Putnam a consequence of which is that typical apples may not have the appearance which we associate with apples.[12] On Putnam's view, to be an apple is to stand in a certain equivalence relation, in this case something like 'the same fruit as', to those things which we commonly identify as apples on the grounds that they have the usual appearances. The equivalence relation is a theoretical relation which is determined independently of the superficial characteristics which make up what we take to be the usual appearances of apples. These characteristics serve to fix the extension of the concept since a thing counts as being in the extension if it has the right relation to the things which have the characteristics. It is in the spirit of the analysis to say that when we describe something as an apple we are saying simply that it is a member of that class whose membership happens to be fixed in this manner. If this view is correct then something could be an apple yet not a member of a kind whose typical members have the usual appearances. This is because typicality is typicality in the class of things which have the right underlying traits—those relevant to the appropriate equivalence relation. Local apples having the usual appearances might turn out not to be typical. Or circumstances may change so that they no longer have the usual appearances.[13] I have already envisaged the possibility that what we think of as the typical visual appearance of apples is not fairly distinctive of apples. That sufficed to make it conceivable that the concept of an apple should be possessed by a group who have no practice of telling that things are apples from their visual appearance. Putnam envisages the rather more dramatic possibility in which apples just do not look the way we take apples typically to look, either because what we think of as the typical look is not typical or because even if apples used to look that way, they no longer do.

I am inclined to think that Putnam is right. The role that the visual appearance of apples has in our practice of applying the concept does not require us to assume that necessarily apples typically have the familiar appearance.

[12] See Putnam (1970, 1975*a*), both repr. in Putnam (1975*b*). Page references are to the latter volume.

[13] Putnam (1970), p. 142.

There is a feature of Putnam's view which can be nicely accommodated in the framework which I am defending. Putnam holds that the familiar appearances of apples contribute to what he calls the stereotype associated with the term. This is a cluster of characteristics which go to make up a conception of typical apples. Putnam suggests that knowing the stereotype is obligatory for those who, as he puts it, acquire the term.[14] He does not have a great deal to say about the nature of this obligation but in the light of the preceding discussion the natural line to take is that the obligation to know, for instance, how apples typically look derives from a current mode of application which *for us* is partially constitutive of mastery of the concept in the broad sense.

It should be said that my own theoretical preferences are rather different from Putnam's. Unlike Putnam I want to link acquiring a term, and thus knowing its meaning, with grasping the concept it expresses. But I also want to distinguish possessing a concept from mastery in the broad sense explained. If we come to think that apples do not typically have or no longer typically have the usual appearance, we should not have to change the concept nor therefore to alter the meaning of the term. We just have to change the relevant mode of application. It would no longer be obligatory to associate apples with what we take to be their typical visual appearance in circumstances in which it is known not to be true that typically they have that appearance.

4.6. *Admissible Contents again*

In the light of the discussion of the last two sections we must consider afresh what sorts of concepts may figure in the descriptive components of the contents of experiences. Clearly the concept of an *F* may have this role if it makes sense to think of an experience as being of an *F*. An experience can be of an *F* only if it makes sense to think of the experience as being *F*-type and such that it seems to the subject that an *F* is there. We can make the second of these conditions more precise in terms of the idea that the concept of an *F* must be experiential.

[14] Putnam (1975*a*), p. 251.

Given the distinction already introduced between broad and narrow senses of 'mastery' we may distinguish between a narrow and a broad conception of the concepts which may figure in the contents of experiences. The narrow conception requires the concepts to be strongly experiential. The broad conception requires only that the concepts should be weakly experiential. Either conception is acceptable. Together they serve to illuminate the relevant intuitions. We are inclined to think that natural-kind concepts can figure in the contents of experiences. This goes along with the thought that it is natural to talk of seeing something as a tiger or as an apple. At the same time we feel that colour concepts, for instance, are more intimately linked to experience than natural-kind concepts. This goes along with the thought that, on a narrower conception of what we can see, we can see that an object is red, but not really see that it is a tiger as opposed to something that merely looks like a tiger.

Thus far I have said nothing about singular contents, that is, contents whose specifications contain singular terms. Are we to allow that experiential contents can be *of Sally* rather than simply *of a woman*? Suppose we regard as Sally-type any experience of a sort which Sally yields. The guiding consideration would then be that an experience could be of Sally if it could be both Sally-type and such that it seems to the subject that Sally is there. We need to make sense of the idea that Sally-type experiences are apt to be such that it seems to the subject that Sally is there. In the non-singular case the aptness of an experience for bearing a certain content depends on its aptness to engage with certain descriptive conceptual capacities. Is there anything similar in the case of singular contents? Well, there is such a thing as knowing who Sally is. But knowing who Sally is cannot require one to be able to recognize Sally via any particular sense-modality. It could easily be the case that Sally is not thus recognizable because she has a twin whose appearance to the modality in question is identical. Yet that would hardly imply that no one could know who Sally is. The situation here is rather like that which we found in connection with the concept of an apple. From the fact that something has the look of an apple one may not infer without further ado that it is an apple. So also from the fact that someone has the look of Sally one may not infer without further ado that she is Sally. And just as a narrow conception of the contents of visual experiences would not allow visual experiences to be of apples, as opposed to being of things having the look of apples, so the natural extension of the narrow conception applied to singular contents would not allow visual experiences to be of Sally as opposed to being of someone having the look of Sally. Nevertheless within a community in which the name 'Sally' is used various things will be taken for granted and used as a basis of communication. Among these might be the proposition that Sally has a fairly distinctive visual appearance. So there will be a way of using the name 'Sally' in response to Sally-type visual experiences the employment of which may be conceived, on a suitably broad conception, as part of what it is to know who Sally is within the community. This broader conception of knowing-who parallels the broader conception of conceptual mastery. It involves capacities which may not be possessed by someone who, in the narrower sense, knows who Sally is. The corresponding broad conception of the contents of visual experiences would allow a visual experience to be of Sally in the community described.

The tolerant attitude which I have adopted towards the question of admissible contents is made possible by the fact that the contents of experiences are not intrinsic. If they were then whether contents of a certain class could be contents of experiences would be determined by the phenomenal character of the experiences. On my account this is not so. Experiences with the same phenomenal character might have different contents depending on differences in the conceptual and other capacities of their respective subjects.

4.7. *Regulative versus Non-Regulative Conceptions of Justification*

As we have seen the approach to justification which I have been developing is regulative in the sense explained in 4.1. It is worth noting before we proceed that it is possible to conceive of regulative constraints on justified belief in ways which would be difficult to reconcile with the view that experiences have a justificatory role. Such a conception can be found in the work of Alvin Goldman who writes as follows:

A regulative system of norms formulates rules to be consciously adopted and followed, for example, precepts or recipes by which an agent should guide his conduct. A nonregulative system of evaluation, by contrast, formulates principles for appraising a performance or trait, or assigning a normative status, but without providing instructions for the *agent* to follow, or apply. They are only principles for an *appraiser* to utilize in judging.[15]

Goldman himself thinks that the norms of justified belief are non-regulative. As he conceives the matter the norms pick out cognitive processes which reliably produce true beliefs. I shall have something to say about his views in the next chapter. Here I just want to underline the fact that Goldman's description of regulative norms does not adequately capture the sorts of regulative constraints which I have identified in this and the preceding two chapters. According to Goldman, a regulative account 'formulates rules to be consciously adopted', rules which are analogous to 'precepts or recipes by which an agent should guide his conduct'. Given these stipulations it is easy to find fault with regulative accounts. All we need do is to focus on *E*-beliefs. Typically when, for instance, you justifiably believe, at least in part on the basis of a current visual experience, that a cup of coffee is on the desk in front of you, you will not have been consciously guided by any 'rules' of an instructional sort such as recipes might be conceived to be. You do not think to yourself that you are having an experience of a cup of coffee, nor that having such an experience is strong evidence that there is a cup of coffee there, nor that your experience should be taken at face value, nor that you may now 'move' to the belief that a cup of coffee is in front of you in accordance with an appropriate rule. So an account of the justification of *E*-beliefs, in terms of the kind of regulative norms described by Goldman, would fail at the first hurdle. The account which I have given does not imply otherwise. I do not suggest that we consciously think of and apply the patterns which guide us in forming and evaluating beliefs. Nevertheless, I do claim that such patterns genuinely govern our thinking in the sense explained earlier.

[15] Goldman (1986), p. 25.

5

Cognitive Capacities and Justification

5.1. *The Enquiry into Human Understanding*

Granted that the conditions on derivatively justified belief set out in Chapters 2 and 4 are along the right lines, a central task of the theory of knowledge must be to describe various types of unconditional reason and the sorts of inference and quasi-inference patterns by which reasons of these types are underwritten. Such a description would yield an account of the corresponding conceptual capacities. It seems plausible that a comprehensive theory of unconditional reasons could be provided using the apparatus introduced earlier. But whether or not that is so, it seems clear in the light of the preceding discussion that epistemology must accord a central role to conceptual analysis, conceived as the analysis of the inference and quasi-inference patterns associated with concepts of various types.

Given the recent history of the subject, talk of conceptual analysis is potentially misleading. In the first place it needs to be stressed that the analysis involved is not concerned solely with epistemological concepts, like those of knowledge and justified belief. A central concern of epistemology must be to examine significant classes of concepts, such as experiential concepts, with a view to reaching an explicit understanding of their inferential and quasi-inferential roles. Recall here that to possess a concept is just to be governed by the patterns by which the concept is individuated, and that means being sensitive to the inferential and quasi-inferential links which instantiate these patterns.

Nor should the analysis which epistemology demands be

conceived as an a priori exercise in any strict sense. Possessing a concept is a matter of having particular conceptual capacities. These capacities are exercised in the management and evaluation of beliefs, and are evidenced by uses of language which express what people believe and why, or which articulate evaluations of beliefs. We become aware of our own uses of language largely by eliciting from ourselves reactions to real or imagined examples. We consider how we should describe certain actual or counterfactual circumstances, we reflect on the reasons we might give for beliefs which we ourselves hold, and by such means we become self-conscious of our conceptual capacities. Notwithstanding the importance of armchair reflection in making our conceptual capacities known to ourselves, it is an empirical matter that we have the capacities we do. Controlled experiments and observations of psychologists from a third-person point of view are relevant in so far as they provide evidence of these capacities. All things considered, the claim that epistemology involves conceptual analysis should not be taken to imply that empirical facts are irrelevant to the conduct of the analysis.[1]

The conception of epistemology which I am defending could be conveniently labelled *conceptualism*, so long as the provisos just noted are borne in mind. I have already stressed (4.1) that the proposed approach to justification is regulative. We are justified in believing that *p* only if in believing that *p* we are guided by the relevant inference and quasi-inference patterns. It follows that conceptualist epistemology must be, in a sense, *psychologistic*. No account of the inferential and quasi-inferential roles of our concepts would be plausible if it were unrealistic from a psychological point of view to suppose that we are actually governed by the patterns which characterize these roles.

This leads us to a question which promises to loom even larger than it does already in theorizing about knowledge. How does the investigation of the conditions of justified belief relate to the investigation of basic cognitive capacities such as perception, memory, the capacity to generalize, and the capacity to acquire concepts? These capacities are basic in that

[1] For some recent reflections on the relation between philosophy and psychology, see the forum on that theme in *Mind and Language*, i. 3–30.

they are native, rather then acquired, and as such are shared by all human beings. Conceptual capacities are also cognitive, but they are not basic because they are acquired.

Obviously, a full understanding of how we acquire knowledge requires an examination of basic cognitive capacities. A full understanding of perception, for instance, would require knowledge of the processes whereby sensory experiences are produced and, through interaction with conceptual capacities, themselves produce beliefs. The investigation of the mechanics of perception has not traditionally fallen within the province of epistemology. But as we have already observed, no account of our concepts would be plausible unless it were psychologically realistic. The account of experiential concepts offered in Chapter 4 would be open to objection if we lacked mechanisms realizing the capacities which the account says that we have. So the conceptualist approach not only allows but demands *rapprochement* between epistemology and psychology. It suggests, however, that if we want to enquire into the mechanics of belief formation we must first have clear models of the conceptual capacities which these mechanisms realize. This constraint derives not from contingent limitations of present theory, but rather from the fact that what makes something a mechanism of belief formation is the fact that it realizes conceptual capacities. There is no way to pick out the mechanisms without a clear view of our conceptual capacities.

There is an alternative approach to epistemology which differs from conceptualism on the matter of how we come by an explicit understanding of the conditions of justified belief. According to conceptualism it is crucial for this task to identify our conceptual capacities in the manner outlined above. The alternative approach has it that we should look rather to our basic cognitive capacities. The rationale for this is the notion that in these capacities lies the clue to how we ought to manage our beliefs. I shall call this general approach *nativism*. One of the things which makes nativism interesting is that it holds out the prospect that epistemology could be revisionary. The thought here is that our acquired methods of belief management and evaluation might be inadequate and that the investigation of our basic cognitive capacities would provide a basis for criticizing these methods and thus much of our actual practice.

In the light of what I have said about conceptualism there is an obvious problem with this approach. Although perception and memory are basic the way they work in acquiring knowledge involves the application of concepts. So we come back to the point that there is no enquiring into how perception and memory function in the acquisition of knowledge without models of our conceptual capacities. Where concept acquisition is concerned essentially the same point applies. We need to have a clear view of the concepts we possess if we are to be in a position to construct plausible models for how concepts are acquired. Nativism seems to be an alternative to conceptualism only if it reverses the proper order of enquiry between basic cognitive capacities and conceptual capacities. I shall pursue this theme throughout this chapter.

It will help to put recent debates in perspective if we recognize that revisionary nativism is deeply rooted in epistemological tradition. The idea that epistemology is a revisionary enterprise and that the warrant for its revisions would emerge from a study of basic cognitive capacities can be found in the work of the classical empiricists, Locke, Berkeley, and Hume. These philosophers had great confidence in the capacity of properly directed enquiry to extend our knowledge, but their confidence was tempered by an appreciation of the extent to which what people think they know is made up of a tissue of traditional opinion, prejudice, superstition, and empty speculation. By determining the limits of knowledge and reasonable enquiry from an investigation of the powers of the understanding, they sought to curb the pretensions of the human mind and remove hindrances to its proper use. A passage from the Introduction to Locke's *Essay* eloquently illustrates the general approach.[2]

For I thought that the first Step towards satisfying several Enquiries, the Mind of Man was very apt to run into, was, to take a Survey of our own Understandings, examine our own Powers, and see to what Things they were adapted. Till that was done I suspected we began at the wrong end and in vain sought for Satisfaction in a quiet and secure Possession of Truths, that most concern'd us, whilst we let loose our Thoughts into the vast Ocean of *Being*, as if all that boundless Extent, were the natural, and undoubted Possession of our Understandings,

[2] The edition is that of P. H. Nidditch, Locke (1979). References in the text are to this edn. giving Book, Chapter, and Section numbers.

wherein there was nothing exempt from its Decisions, or that escaped its Comprehension. Thus Men, extending their Enquiries beyond their Capacities, and letting their Thoughts wander into those depths, where they can find no sure Footing; 'tis no Wonder, that they raise Questions, and multiply Disputes, which never coming to any clear Resolution, are proper only to continue and increase their Doubts, and to confirm them at last in perfect Scepticism. (I. i. 7)

As we shall see, it is clear that the capacities which Locke wishes to investigate are basic. He is undoubtedly concerned to understand various types of acquired conceptual capacity, but his treatment of these is guided by a theory of concept acquisition which places significant constraints on the sorts of concepts we can be said to possess and thus on the scope of reasonable enquiry. Locke, like other classical epistemologists, believed that the principles of sound enquiry were not widely enough appreciated and were commonly flouted in both science and religion. His epistemology, grounded in an examination of the native powers of the understanding, was meant to show what the appropriate constraints are, steer people away from unsound reasoning and judgement, and set enquiry on the right course into the 'vast ocean of Being'. It would thus have a significant revisionary function in so far as it would show people where reforms are needed in their thinking.

In the next section we shall take a closer look at what Locke has to say paying special attention to his view of the relationship between how our concepts are acquired and how our enquiries should be directed. In the section following I shall take up some neglected themes from Hume. As well as illuminating the work of these philosophers, this historical excursus will serve to highlight the general difficulty for nativism which I have identified.

5.2. *Locke on Concept Acquisition*

Much of what Locke has to say about ideas is clearly about what we would call concepts. There are difficulties, however, for any straightforward identification of Lockian ideas with concepts. For instance, if ideas are concepts what should we make of the distinction between particular and general ideas? Locke thinks it evident that children have a particular idea of their mothers. The idea is associated with a name like 'mamma' used for the single individual who is the child's mother. After acquaintance with a number of human beings besides mother, children frame a general idea of a man which applies to all who are in various respects like those human beings they have encountered. As Locke puts it,

> *they come to have a general Name*, and a general *Idea*. Wherein they make nothing new, but only leave out of the complex *Idea* they had of *Peter* and *James, Mary* and *Jane*, that which is peculiar to each, and retain only what is common to them all. (III. iii. 7)

I think it is fairly clear that particular ideas, for Locke, are images.[3] So far as the ideas of sensation are concerned, they are sensory images, which is to say, sensory experiences, or replays of sensory experiences,[4] or sensory imaginings. This view of the matter fits what Locke says about the particular ideas of children.

> The *Ideas* of the Nurse, and the Mother, are well framed in their Minds; and, like Pictures of them there, represent only those Individuals. (III. iii. 7)

Elsewhere Locke explicitly regards sensations as ideas (II. viii. 8), and, as we shall see in a moment, his account of the genesis of general ideas requires particular ideas to be something like images. Although Locke is not careful about the matter, much of what he says requires particular ideas to be image types rather than tokens.[5] For instance, Locke makes it clear that we can retain particular ideas in the mind even when their tokens do not occur as conscious episodes. To have an idea thus stored in the mind is nothing other than the capacity to call its tokens into consciousness realizing that one has had such tokens before (II. x. 2). Since you can recall an idea that you had previously, these ideas must be repeatables. A similar story applies, though less plausibly, to the ideas of reflection. Particular ideas of reflection would be repeatable images obtained from perception of the operations of our own minds.

[3] Ayers (1986) explores in some detail the role of images in Locke's account of thought.

[4] On the idea of replaying experiences, see 4.2 and Lyons (1986).

[5] See Ayers (1986), p. 7.

A further complication must be noted. Sensory images have a complexity which is reflected in the multiplicity of non-equivalent ways in which they may be described. This point is just an extension of one which has been prominent in the discussion of experience in earlier chapters. One and the same experience may be of the type produced by something white, of the type produced by something round, of the type produced by something yellow and square, and so forth. Locke recognizes that a particular idea which a child might have of its mother would have this complexity. Strictly speaking, since a complex particular idea would be an image type of an entire scene, it is inaccurate to speak of the particular idea which the child has of its mother. What is thus loosely described is in fact a whole range of complex particular ideas of the mother in various settings and attitudes. A simple particular idea would be a feature of an image type, for example the sort of feature which would normally be produced by a red thing. The boy who comes to form the general idea of a man 'leaves out' of the complex ideas of his mother, brothers, and friends those features 'peculiar to each' and attends to those common to all which are relevant to the general idea.

Particular ideas are not well suited to play the role of concepts if for no other reason than that they 'represent' only particular individuals. General descriptive concepts apply, or at least could in principle apply, to many individuals and this is what Locke takes to be the function of general ideas. We may certainly think of Locke as having a theory of concepts and of concept acquisition in so far as he has a theory of general ideas and how we come by them.

Locke's theory of concept acquisition is an empiricist one according to which all concepts are acquired from perception, understood in broad terms to include not only sense-perception, but also reflection, the inner perception of the workings of our own minds (II. i). The distinction between simple and complex also applies to concepts, though Locke fails to note that complexity of concepts is very different from complexity of images. Complexity in concepts has to do with their being definable in terms of other concepts. Simple concepts are indefinable (III. iv. 4 ff.). Complexity in images is multiplicity of features. Locke's simple particular ideas are features of images which do not break down into other features. The simplest concepts we can acquire, on Locke's view, are of properties which sensory or inner perceptions convey to us, and these form a fairly restricted class. Thus, for example, we acquire concepts of qualities such as whiteness, heat, softness, and sweetness, by perceiving, in the appropriate sense-modality, things which have these qualities. Locke thinks that we also acquire simple concepts of solidity, extension, figure, number, motion, and rest, in essentially the same way, though in their case more than one modality is involved. So far as reflection is concerned we are supposed to acquire concepts of acts of the mind such as thinking and willing, and their various 'modes' as we perceive particular instances of such acts. All our other concepts are supposed to be explicable in terms of simple concepts. The upshot is that all concepts result from experience since experience furnishes the mind with the materials for all the concepts we are capable of possessing.

At the heart of Locke's theory is an account of how perception results in the acquisition of simple concepts. Consider the concept of being red. According to Locke, we are able to acquire this concept because we have various complex particular ideas which share that feature which is usually produced by red things, the simple idea of red. The process whereby we arrive at the concept of being red from these complex particular ideas is what Locke calls *abstraction* (II. xi. 9 ff.). Having obtained complex particular ideas from red things, the simple particular idea of red which is their common element comes to be representative of everything having the quality of being red. To have the general idea of being red is to be able to 'use' the simple particular idea so that it represents all red things.

This story is notoriously puzzling. One of the problems is that Locke often seems to conceive of abstraction as a process which requires the subject to survey particular ideas. If particular ideas are images of one kind or another this is implausible. In contemplating objects we may notice and compare their features, but would not in general consider features of the experiences which they yield. Locke is well aware of the difference between ideas in the mind and qualities of objects, as the following passage illustrates.

> Whatsoever the Mind perceives in it self, or is the immediate object of Perception, Thought, or Understanding, that I call *Idea*; and the power to produce any *Idea* in our mind, I call *Quality* of the Subject wherein that power is. (II. viii. 8)

But he also recognizes that sometimes he uses the term 'idea' for qualities. Shortly after the passage just quoted he says, 'if I speak [of ideas] sometimes, as in the things themselves, I would be understood to mean those Qualities in the Objects which produce them in us'. So it should come as no surprise that within the space of a sentence he can speak in a manner which suggests both that abstraction involves noticing qualities shared by objects and that it involves noticing features of what is conveyed to the mind when objects are observed.

> Thus the same Colour being observed to day in Chalk or Snow, which the Mind yesterday received from Milk, it considers that Appearance alone, makes it a representative of all of that kind . . . (II. xi. 9)

I do not think it can be denied that Locke holds to the mistaken view that concept acquisition involves noticing features of experiences. But his account of abstraction does seem to imply three more plausible theses which are independent of that mistaken view. The first is that we acquire simple concepts of sensation by exposure to instances of the concept. Thus we acquire the concept of redness through exposure to red things. The second is that to have a simple concept of sensation is to be able to recognize instances on the basis of current experience. The third is that experience-based recognition of instances is made possible by the fact that the experiences which instances yield have a common feature. In the case of the concept of redness this common feature would be what Locke thinks of as the simple particular idea of redness.

Another problem is to understand in what sense simple particular ideas come to represent all things. The result of the process is clear to this extent. We come to have a general idea of being red which applies to all red things and not just to those we have contemplated. The trouble is that Locke seems to think of a general idea as a particular idea which has a certain representative role. Given the sharp distinction which we make between concepts and experiences this seems an odd account of anything that we would regard as a concept. Nevertheless, as I have just suggested, at least part of what Locke wants to say is that to have the general idea of being red is to be able to recognize red things in virtue of having a complex particular idea which has a feature usually produced by red things. This makes it natural to conceive of the representative role of that feature as consisting in its being the common feature of experiences in virtue of which we notice redness in things.

The mode of acquisition of the concept of redness seems to be for Locke the model for all simple concepts relating to a single sense-modality. There are also simple concepts relating to diverse senses. Locke lists the ideas of extension, figure, motion, and rest. Where these are concerned the only departure from the model would seem to be that to have such a concept is to be able to judge something to have the property in question when it produces an appropriate experience in one or other of the relevant modalities.

The proposed account of abstraction commits Locke to the following *Applicability thesis*: Simple concepts of sensation are applicable (i.e. may legitimately be applied) only to objects which yield experiences having an appropriate feature. To have such a concept is just to be able to apply it in response to appropriate experiences to objects which yield these experiences. As we shall see in a moment the Applicability thesis is important for Locke's treatment of real essences. Before we come to that it is of some interest to consider a stronger thesis to which Locke might seem to be committed. This is that a thing can be an instance of a simple concept of sensation only if it has the power to yield experiences having an appropriate feature. This *Instance thesis* should not be conflated with the Applicability thesis. The latter gives a condition for our taking something to be an instance of a concept. The former gives a condition on a thing's being an instance of a concept. Yet there is a plausible line of thought connecting the two theses.

As I noted in Chapter 4, although we have a practice of telling that a thing is an apple from its visual appearance, our concept of an apple leaves room for the possibility that there are apples which do not have the usual visual appearance and thus would not yield experiences of the type which we think of as apple-type. By contrast, given the Applicability thesis, Lockian simple concepts of sensation would not be applicable to a thing unless that thing yielded experiences of the appropriate type. But now, the constraints on the applicability of a concept fix the conditions for something's being an instance of the concept. So the Instance thesis holds if the Applicability thesis does.

Locke does accept the Applicability thesis. It is at the basis of his discussion of real essences, as we shall see presently. There are passages which might suggest that he accepts the Instance thesis too. If qualities, as Locke states (II. viii. 8), are powers to produce ideas, it would seem that simple qualities corresponding to simple concepts of sensation would be powers to produce ideas of those qualities. The ideas in question could be nothing other than complex particular ideas, that is, sensory experiences yielded by things having the quality in question. So to have a quality of this type would just be to have the power to yield experiences of the appropriate sort. However, Locke certainly does not consistently hold to the Instance thesis. He clearly envisages that the minute unobservable parts of matter have qualities like extension, figure, and motion (II. viii. 9; cf. IV. xvi. 12) which Locke regards as corresponding to simple concepts of sensation. It is not true of such minute parts that they yield experiences of the appropriate sort. A minute particle might be round, and might be implicated in the production of experiences of something round, but such experiences would not be such as could form the basis of a judgement that the particle is round, as opposed to the body of which it is a part. The Instance thesis is clearly implausible so far as concepts of extension, figure, and motion are concerned.

It might be wondered whether the Instance thesis is consistent with Locke's distinction between primary and secondary qualities. After all Locke means to distinguish secondary qualities from primary when he says that the former are powers to produce sensations in us. So it might look as if the distinction would collapse if the Instance thesis were true.

Locke makes two principal claims about the distinction. The first is that whereas primary qualities are inseparable from bodies, secondary qualities are mere powers to produce sensations in us in virtue of the primary qualities possessed by the minute parts of the body in question (II. viii. 9 f.). The second is that whereas the '*Ideas of primary Qualities* of Bodies, *are*

Resemblances of them, and their Patterns do really exist in the Bodies themselves', the ideas of secondary qualities '*have no resemblance* of them at all' (II. viii. 15).

The second claim, which might be called the Resemblance thesis, admits of two distinct interpretations depending on how literally we take the notion of resemblance. It might be taken to imply that whereas to our idea of extension there *corresponds* a quality, extension, which bodies really have, to our idea of redness there is no corresponding quality, redness, which bodies really have. But then it is difficult to square this with the view that redness is a power in bodies, a power which bodies presumably really have to produce sensations in us. On the other hand, the notion of resemblance may be taken more literally. The Resemblance thesis could be read to imply that whereas the idea, the particular idea, which a body produces in us in virtue of being extended resembles the quality extension in bodies, the idea which red things produce in us in virtue of being red does not resemble the quality redness in bodies. I suspect that Locke's own understanding of the Resemblance thesis conflates these readings. On neither reading is the thesis at all plausible. It is just mistaken to suppose that simple particular ideas, conceived as repeatable features of experiences, are in the running for either resembling or failing to resemble the qualities of bodies in any literal sense. Experiences of extended bodies do not have a feature which resembles extension.[6]

The correspondence reading runs into difficulties if secondary qualities are powers which bodies really have. The difficulties relate to Locke's first claim about the primary–secondary quality distinction: that whereas primary qualities are inseparable from bodies, secondary qualities are powers to produce sensations in us. Locke seems to gloss the idea that primary qualities are inseparable from bodies by saying that they are in bodies whether or not they are perceived. But then the same would be true of secondary qualities in so far as they are conceived as powers to produce experiences in us. I think the problem here is due to the fact that Locke tends to identify secondary qualities

[6] That experiences of *F* things are not *F* experiences is a pervasive and important theme of Sellars's work. See Sellars (1963,1968). Peacocke's account of sensational properties is designed to accommodate the point. See above, 1.7.

with features of experiences. For instance, he thinks that the quality whiteness stands to the body which we call white as pain stands to something which produces pain in us (II. viii. 17). That is why he can think of secondary qualities as not really being in bodies. For pain is not in the body which produces it and so, by the analogy, whiteness would not be in the bodies we call white. This way of thinking of whiteness fits well with the correspondence reading of the Resemblance thesis, but, unfortunately, is inconsistent with the view that whiteness is a power to produce experiences having a certain feature.

It is interesting to note that a primary–secondary quality distinction could be preserved even if all qualities are conceived as powers to produce experiences in us. A quality *Q* would be a primary quality if and only if it is a power in bodies to produce experiences (complex particular ideas) which have a certain feature (a simple particular idea) *Q*', which is characteristic of experiences produced by bodies having *Q*, and which resembles *Q*. A quality *Q* would be a secondary quality if and only if it is a power to produce experiences which have a feature *Q*' which is characteristic of experiences produced by bodies having *Q*, but which does not resemble *Q*. This way of taking the distinction makes the literal reading of the Resemblance thesis central with the consequent problems which that involves. Note, however, that there is no incompatibility between this conception of the primary–secondary quality distinction and the Instance thesis.

Our main concern is with how by understanding a basic cognitive capacity, concept acquisition, we are supposed to gain insight into what we may know or justifiably believe. In this connection Locke's discussions of our ideas of substances are crucial and will serve to illustrate the relevance of the theses about concepts and qualities which I have just considered.

Locke holds that the concepts we attach to substance words like 'gold' pertain to perceptible properties of the things to which they apply. We think of gold as 'a Body yellow, of a certain weight, malleable, fusible, and fixed' (III. vi. 2). These properties make up the nominal essence of gold as opposed to its real essence. The real essence of a substance is its internal constitution and this accounts for the properties which make up its nominal essence. The problem, Locke thinks, is that philosophers tend to suppose that they have an idea of the real essence of a substance when all they have is an idea of its nominal essence. But Locke goes much further than this for he thinks that there are difficulties in the notion that we could ever come by an idea of the real essence of a substance.

Part of the difficulty derives from Locke's view of what it would be to have a concept, a general idea, of the real essence of a substance. Such an idea would be complex and thus would be made up of simple ideas. But there is a problem about the applicability of simple general ideas to the minute parts which make up the internal constitution of a substance, a problem which stems from the intimate relation between general and particular ideas consequent upon the way in which general ideas are acquired. If the Applicability thesis is true then we are not in a position to apply simple general ideas of sensation to unobservable particles or systems of particles. And if that is true then we are in no position to obtain complex general ideas of the internal constitutions of things. Hence the significance of the proposition that '[o]ur Faculties carry us no farther towards the knowledge and distinction of Substances, than a Collection of those sensible *Ideas*, which we observe in them' (III. vi. 9). Moreover, if the Instance thesis is true then not only are we in no position to judge that minute unobservable particles or systems of such particles have such-and-such qualities; these particles or systems of particles will not be instances of these qualities either. It should be remembered, however, that Locke himself does not hold consistently to the Instance thesis.

There are other strands in Locke's thought about real essences which are less germane to our present concerns. For instance, Locke holds that if we had a concept, a complex general idea, of the real essence of a substance 'then the Properties we discover in that Body, would depend on that complex *Idea*, and be deducible from it, and their necessary connexion with it be known; as all the Properties of a Triangle depend on, and as far as they are discoverable, are deducible from the complex *Idea* of three Lines, including a Space' (II. xxxi. 6). Although we know that gold is heavy, malleable and so on, "tis impossible we should know what other Qualities result from, or are incompatible with the . . . Constitution of the insensible parts of Gold . . .' (IV. iii. 11). No more can we know how the internal constitution of gold relates to its nominal essence. Locke concludes that the generalizations we make about the observable properties of a substance must be based on observation of samples of the substance. We can make probable conjectures about as yet unknown properties, but we cannot know them to be true since 'the highest Probability, amounts not to Certainty; without which, there can be no true Knowledge' (IV. iii. 14). This last conclusion, it should be noted, is a special assumption about knowledge which appears to be independent of the theory of concept acquisition.

That theories of knowledge must take account of our actual cognitive capacities ought to go without saying. As I have stressed already, plausible formulations of the constraints on justified belief must be psychologically realistic. Locke, Berkeley, and Hume realized this, and it is an important consideration for naturalistic epistemologists of the present day. This granted, it remains an open question whether an examination of capacities, such as concept acquisition, can yield an epistemology of the sort envisaged by Locke. The project, in general terms, is to derive an account of how we ought to manage and evaluate beliefs from consideration of basic capacities, the powers of the understanding. It is central to Locke's working out of the project that the study of concept acquisition discloses significant general strictures on the kinds of concepts we can be said to possess and on the conditions of their applicability. Thus where simple concepts of sensation are concerned the account of abstraction yields the Applicability thesis which in turn accounts for the limits which Locke discerns on enquiry into real essences.

The Applicability thesis is open to objection if for no other reason than that it yields the Instance thesis given the plausible assumption that the conditions of the Applicability of a concept fix the conditions for a thing to be an instance of the concept. If this is right then although Locke holds that minute particles have extension and motion his theory of abstraction implies an account of the concepts of extension and motion which leaves no room for that possibility.

For the strategic concerns of this chapter it is important to appreciate the source of Locke's difficulties. The main problem, I suspect, is the idea that by taking a survey of our experiences both sensory and 'inner' and of the sorts of properties which they can have, we can appreciate what concepts are available to us and the conditions under which they may be applied to things by us. In Locke's framework this idea is worked out in terms of two principal theses. The first, is that all concepts are either simple or derive from simple concepts. The second is that which simple concepts we can have is determined by intrinsic properties of experiences, Locke's simple particular ideas. But the idea is wrong in principle. Our grasp of the character of our experiences depends on the repertoire of concepts which we apply to the environment. This is true whether we describe phenomenal character in terms of the *F*-type typology or in terms of Peacocke's sensational properties. Experiences themselves do not provide us with a check on the kinds of concepts which can be applied on their basis.

To understand the nature of our concepts we have to reflect on the ways in which we form, maintain, and evaluate beliefs. This is what reveals our conceptual capacities and thus illuminates the conditions of justified belief. As I suggested in 5.1, if we want to enquire into our basic cognitive capacities in a manner which is relevant to a concern with justified belief then we must first be clear about our conceptual capacities. Locke reverses the proper order of enquiry. He proceeds as if we could determine what conceptual capacities we do and could have through enquiry into how concepts are acquired. He adopts this strategy because he mistakenly thinks that the character of our experiences fixes what concepts we can have.

5.3. *Hume on Generalization*

The concerns which inform Hume's writings are very much those of Locke. In the Introduction to the *Treatise of Human Nature* he writes,[7]

> Even *Mathematics, Natural Philosophy, and Natural Religion*, are in some measure dependent on the science of Man; since they lie under the cognizance of men, and are judged of by their powers and faculties. 'Tis impossible to tell what changes and improvements we might make in

[7] References in the text are to the Selby-Bigge edn., Hume (1888), giving Book, Part, Section, and, where appropriate, page numbers.

these sciences were we thoroughly acquainted with the extent and force of human understanding, and cou'd explain the nature of the ideas we employ, and of the operations we perform in our reasonings. (Intro. xix)

Hume proposes, therefore, to apply to the study of human nature, including our cognitive capacities, the experimental method which had proved successful in the best of recent science, that of Newton. Initially, this might seem an odd procedure if the aim was to improve science having first learned about our cognitive capacities. But Hume's aim is to use the best scientific method to understand how that can and must be the best method. I find it difficult to see how one could read the *Treatise* and suppose that this is not Hume's intention. If it is, then Hume is, undoubtedly, a nativist epistemologist with revisionary aims. There arises the question of how his normative epistemological concerns relate to his use of the 'experimental method'.

A good starting-point is a famous passage in the *Treatise*.

Nature, by an absolute and uncontroulable necessity has determin'd us to judge as well as to breathe and feel; . . . Whoever has taken the pains to refute the cavils of . . . *total* scepticism, has really disputed without an antagonist, and endeavour'd by arguments to establish a faculty, which nature has antecedently implanted in the mind, and render'd unavoidable. (I. IV. i. 183)

The faculty of which Hume speaks is a basic cognitive capacity whereby patterns in past experience yield dispositions to form beliefs of certain types on having sensory impressions of certain types. For example, we are so disposed that on hearing a knocking sound at the study door we believe that someone wishes to see us. This disposition is essentially a habit of inference which, according to Hume's principles, is inculcated by past experience and in particular by a pattern whereby an experience of a knocking sound at a door is constantly, or at least very regularly, conjoined with an experience of people wishing to see us. In the quoted passage Hume is saying that the faculty which converts past experience of the sort described into dispositions of the sort described is implanted in us by nature and that its exercise is unavoidable. Hume also believes that no amount of argument will establish that our adoption of inferential habits by the suggested mechanism is justified. This is the force of a remark made in an earlier section of the *Treatise* which may stand for many.

> Reason can never satisfy us that the existence of any one object does ever imply that of another; so that when we pass from the impression of one to the idea or belief of another, we are not determin'd by reason, but by custom or a principle of association. (I. III. vii. 97)

It is crucially important not to read more into this passage than is actually there. Hume is concerned with how we come by habits of inference and thus how we come to make particular inferences. The claim is not that the acquisition of habits of inference and the making of particular inferences is irrational. It is simply that we cannot by argument establish that we are justified in proceeding as we do. Hume's defence of this claim rests on his classification of modes of reasoning into two types, demonstrative and matter-of-fact. Demonstrative reasoning applies only to conclusions whose negation is impossible (I. III. vi; I. IV. ii). Matter-of-fact reasoning presupposes that we may make inferences in accordance with habits induced by past experience and so cannot establish the legitimacy of proceeding in this way. So either way reason cannot justify our acquiring, and inferring in accordance with, habits of inference of the sort in question. However, it does not follow that the acquisition of such habits and the making of such inferences is irrational. To draw that conclusion would require the assumption that a practice is irrational unless its soundness is established by argument, and there is no reason to suppose that Hume accepted or should have accepted any such assumption.

Hume is not simply concerned to offer, so to speak, an anatomy and physiology of human understanding. That is to say, he is not simply concerned with the structure of the mind and how it works. He is also concerned to develop a model of justification, as his most renowned polemical remark indicates.

> If we take in our hand any volume; of divinity or school metaphysics, for instance; let us ask, *Does it contain any abstract reasoning concerning quantity or number?* No. *Does it contain any experimental reasoning concerning matter of fact and existence?* No. Commit it then to the flames: for it can contain nothing but sophistry and illusion.

This occurs right at the end of the first *Enquiry*[8] and it forms in effect the leitmotif of the *Dialogues Concerning Natural Religion.*[9] In the latter work Hume clearly presupposes that a sound argument for the existence of God would have to be either demonstrative (abstract) or matter-of-fact (experimental) and tries to show that no sound argument of either type could establish that God exists. The entire work constitutes a critique of natural theology as his essay on miracles constitutes, in effect, a critique of revelation-based theology. Both critiques rely on a model of justified belief. The evidence that Hume was concerned to develop such a model is not confined to the first *Enquiry* and the *Dialogues*. In Book I of the *Treatise* he offers some general rules 'by which to judge of causes and effects' (I. iii. xv). These are rules whereby we may come to know and thus justifiably believe that events are causally related.

There remains, though, a serious question of how on Hume's general principles there can be such a thing as justified belief and how we can discern the constraints on justified belief. The basic problem is to see how the application of the experimental method to the operations of the understanding can tell us about the general principles which determine which of our beliefs are justified. Supposing Hume is right in thinking that nature has implanted in us a faculty whereby past experience generates habits of inference, how are we to tell which habits are sound and which unsound? Hume undoubtedly felt the force of these questions for he explicitly discusses the problem in a rather neglected section of the *Treatise* (I. III. xiii) which deals with what he calls 'unphilosophical probability'.

In the section concerned Hume discusses various factors which can lead us to suppose certain sorts of proposition probable. These probabilities are called unphilosophical because the factors in question are not ones which philosophers would regard as providing a sound basis for accepting the propositions in question. Hume offers examples which are particularly germane to the matter in hand. They concern '*general rules*, which we rashly form to ourselves, and which are the source of what we properly call PREJUDICE' (I. III. xiii. 146). Hume's specific examples of prejudice are that an Irishman cannot have

[8] Hume (1902), p. 165.
[9] Hume (1970).

wit and a Frenchman cannot have solidity. In this context general rules are simply universal generalizations. Accepting any such generalization is tantamount to having a habit of inference. Hume explains the acquisition of habits such as this in terms of our tendency to generalize too hastily by giving too much weight to insignificant analogies. He says, '[W]e transfer our experience in past instances to objects which are resembling, but are not exactly the same with those concerning which we have had experience' (I. iii. xiii. 147). Here we are operating in accordance with what might be called a higher-order general rule, a rule for acquiring rules. But the higher-order rule is crude and unreliable because it leads us to form generalizations without due regard to the difference between 'accidental circumstances' and 'efficacious causes' (I. iii. xiii. 149). Hume presumably thinks the prejudice about Frenchmen is acquired in this way. We encounter a few people who lack solidity (perish the thought), and who happen to be French, and this leads us to suppose that all Frenchmen have this unfortunate defect. What we fail to realize is that being French has nothing to do with the lack of solidity of the Frenchmen we have met. It is an accidental circumstance.

Hume's account is fairly obviously inadequate. For one thing it fails to acknowledge the extent to which prejudice is induced and reinforced by education. (Indeed, it is a defect of Hume's general treatment of how we come by habits of inference that it frequently ignores the role which he himself accords to education in *Treatise* I. iii. ix.) The point upon which I wish to focus, however, is independent of the detailed treatment of prejudice. It is that if some habits of inference are to be supposed sound and others unsound then Hume is going to have to distinguish between good and bad methods of acquiring such habits and thus between good and bad higher-order general rules. This is precisely what Hume does when he distinguishes between general rules which are 'extensive and constant' and those which are 'capricious and uncertain', reckoning the former to judgement and the latter to imagination. We should not be misled by the fact that Hume often uses the term 'imagination' for that faculty whereby the mind makes a transition from one state to another in accordance with learned uniformities. The essential point is that where Hume opposes imagination to judgement he has in mind imagination operating in accordance with rules which are 'capricious and uncertain' as it does in generating prejudice. The exercise of judgement also involves imagination, but this time operating in accordance with rules which are 'extensive and constant'. The following passage makes this clear.

When an object appears, that resembles any cause in very considerable circumstances, the imagination naturally carries us to a lively conception of the usual effect, tho' the object be different in the most material and most efficacious circumstances from that cause. Here is the first influence of general rules. But when we take a review of this act of the mind, and compare it with the more general and authentic operations of the understanding, we find it to be of an irregular nature, and destructive of all the most establish'd principles of reasoning; which is the cause of our rejecting it. This is a second influence of general rules and implies the condemnation of the former. (I. III. xiii. 149–50)

The suggestion is that through a review of the operations of the understanding we come to appreciate that the way we acquire prejudices conflicts with established principles of reasoning, such as those which Hume formulates in *Treatise* I. III. xv to 'regulate our judgment concerning causes and effects'.

There seem to be two levels in Hume's thinking about these matters. At one level he is concerned to describe the operations of the mind and in particular to account for the acquisition of habits of inference and of the beliefs which we acquire by the exercise of these habits. At this level general rules are simply laws in accordance with which the mind operates. At another level Hume is concerned to give some account of the role in our thinking of principles which are germane to the evaluation of beliefs and modes of reasoning. It is in connection with this level that he speaks of 'authentic operations of the understanding' and 'establish'd principles of reasonings'.

The picture which Hume presents is something like this. We have a faculty whereby we form habits of inference on the basis of past experience. These are the habits in which our acceptance of universal generalizations consists. Some, like those corresponding to the prejudices noted earlier, are unreliable in that, as often as not, they take us from truths to falsehoods. Others reliably, if not infallibly, take us from truths to truths. However, reflection shows that we acquire some inferential habits in ways which violate sound higher-order general rules, the 'establish'd principles of reasoning', in particular those by which 'we learn to distinguish the accidental circumstances from the efficacious causes'.

But (i) what makes a rule an established principle of reasoning and (ii) how can we tell which rules enjoy that status? So far as (ii) is concerned Hume tells us that 'these rules are form'd on the nature of our understanding, and on our experience of its operations in the judgments we form concerning objects' (I. III. xiii. 149). The reflective exercise whereby we come to discriminate between good and bad general rules, and reckon the former to judgement and the latter to imagination, is conceived as an extension of the experimental method of reasoning to acts of the mind. This naturally raises the question of how such an exercise can enable us to discern what are, in effect, norms of justified belief.[10] This is where Hume's answer to (i) comes in, or, at least, an answer which might be constructed from his cursory remarks on the topic. Hume does explicitly say that the rules which we attribute to judgement are 'extensive and constant'. I think he is feeling his way towards the idea that some ways of acquiring those habits of inference which correspond to the acceptance of generalizations are 'general and authentic operations of the understanding' just because they reliably issue in the acquisition of habits of inference which are themselves reliable. If this is what he thinks it provides a clue to how he conceives the status of 'established principles of reasoning'. These would be higher-order rules enjoining us to employ those operations which are reliable in the way indicated.

This interpretation explains how Hume could suppose that the application of the experimental method to the understanding, and, in particular, to the basic cognitive capacity we have for generalizing, could disclose constraints on justified belief. If the hallmark of a justified belief is its being acquired by authentic operations of the understanding, and if we can determine which operations are authentic experimentally, by finding out which reliably issue in reliable generalizations, then

[10] Compare Buchdahl (1969), p. 347: '[T]erms like "more general and authentic" should really have no place in this context, where we expected our rules of reasoning to be built upon a merely natural and instinctive basis.' This judgement, I think, is premature. See below.

the experimental study of the understanding will disclose which norms we should adopt.

Read in this way Hume offers the prospect of an approach to epistemology which is nativist in so far as it seeks to understand the constraints on justified belief via the investigation of our basic cognitive faculties.[11] I shall not attempt to offer a detailed criticism of his treatment of our generalizing faculty. Hume seems to me to be profoundly right in two respects, first, in that he recognizes the futility of seeking reasons for engaging in the practice of forming generalizations from past experience, secondly, in that he saw that some ways of forming generalizations are better than others. There is a serious question, though, concerning the plausibility of the idea that the constraints on justified belief are disclosed to us through a review of the operations of the understanding of the sort which Hume appears to envisage. One very basic problem concerns the idea that we could conduct such a review while being ignorant of what constitutes good reasons for empirical generalizations. The aim is to examine ways in which we have formed generalizations in the past. So, asked why you thought that all *F*s are *G*, you might point out that every *F* you had encountered was *G*. Most likely you did not explicitly reason that since every *F* you had encountered was *G* it was highly probable that all *F*s are *G*. So your understanding of how you came to hold the generalization would probably not derive from your recollection of an actual inference. It would derive rather from your now appreciating the relevance of positive and negative instances to generalizations, an appreciation which is partially constitutive of your grasp of the universal quantifier. You would rely on this grasp in making conjectures about the kind of operation of the understanding which led to your accepting the generalization in question. But in that case a review of the operations of the understanding of the Humean sort cannot disclose the constraints on the justified formation of generalizations. On the contrary, in order to conduct the review you already require to have a grasp of the relevant constraints.

To press home this last point we need only reflect further on the problem which engages Hume in the section 'Of

[11] If this interpretation is correct then Hume is a precursor of modern reliability theorists of justification such as Goldman. See below, 5.4.

unphilosophical probability'. Having encountered positive instances and no negative instances does not suffice to make a generalization acceptable. That is why Hume appeals to general rules of the understanding. Again, though, we should ask how we know what else is relevant. Suppose you once caught a few fish which you had never encountered before and found good to eat. You drew the conclusion that all fish of this kind are good to eat. Being interested in matters ecological you also noted that all the fish which you caught of this kind were male. Needless to say you did not draw the conclusion that all such fish are male. A review of the understanding which is to meet Hume's requirements should reveal why this last generalization is unsound while the former is sound. But, again, in order to get a grip on how your mind actually operated in the circumstance in which you drew the one conclusion but not the other you have to read in your present understanding of the constraints relevant to the generalizations in question. This understanding would have to derive from reflection on the relevant kinds of conceptual competence operating against a background of substantive beliefs about the world. Thus you would draw on background beliefs to the effect that good eating quality is fairly constant across a kind of fish, while gender obviously is not. So once again the Humean review cannot disclose the constraints on justification for we need to know what these are in order to conduct it.

It is extremely important to appreciate that I am not criticizing Hume for confusing factual psychology with normative matters.[12] Hume is much more sophisticated in this matter than he is usually taken to be, and if I am right, he is, at least, heading in the direction of an account of how psychology relates to epistemology. My criticism is rather that Hume wrongly supposes that we can come to an appreciation of justificational constraints by studying the operation of basic capacities. We shall return to this theme shortly. Before we do, and in keeping with the central concerns of this book, I shall take a look at the implications of Hume's treatment of generalization for the justification of *E*-beliefs, that is, beliefs about the present environment based on current experience.

[12] This sort of criticism has been directed towards Hume. See e.g. Passmore (1968), p. 18 ff., and Bennett (1971), pp. 230 ff.

In Treatise I. iv. ii, Hume tries to apply his general theory of matter-of-fact reasoning to *E*-beliefs, the central thought being that if we could base beliefs about present objects on current experience then there would have to be well-founded generalizations connecting the occurrence of experiences of certain types with the presence of objects of certain corresponding types. However, Hume thinks that this approach does not work. Part of the difficulty which he encounters has to do with an aspect of his thought about generalization which I have ignored so far but which is highly germane to the central concerns of this book. It comes out in a passage in which Hume explains why matter-of-fact reasoning cannot properly assure us that there are bodies which are distinct from our experiences and which continue to exist when not perceived.

> [S]ince nothing is ever really present to the mind, besides its own perceptions, 'tis not only impossible, that any habit shou'd ever be acquir'd otherwise than by the regular succession of these perceptions, but also that any habit shou'd ever exceed that degree of regularity. Any degree, therefore, of regularity in our perceptions, can never be a foundation for us to infer a greater degree of regularity in some objects, which are not perceiv'd; since this supposes a contradiction, *viz.* a habit acquir'd by what was never present to the mind. But 'tis evident, that whenever we infer the continu'd existence of the objects of sense from their coherence, and the frequency of their union, 'tis in order to bestow on the objects a greater regularity than what is observ'd in our mere perceptions. (I. iv. ii. 197)

When Hume is not perplexed by problems of the external world he is happy to talk as if our habits of inference are acquired on the basis of observations of conjunctions of events or conjunctions of properties in objects, where these events and objects are conceived to be in the world around us. The habits take us from an experience (impression) of some event or state of affairs to an idea, in effect an expectation, that some distinct event or state of affairs will occur or will be found to occur. However, the passage quoted, and many others in *Treatise* I. iv. ii, show that Hume sometimes thinks of experiences (impressions) as being themselves objects of perception. This, disastrously, leads him to conceive of habits of inference as if they took us from a belief to the effect that we are having an experience of a certain sort to an expectation that we will have an experience of another sort. If this were right then no habit of inference could take us from a belief that we are having an experience of a certain sort to a belief that an object of a certain sort is before us, for this would require there to be habits 'acquir'd by what was never present to the mind', namely a conjunction of an experience and a present object.

Hume realizes that given this view of the matter there is a serious problem not just about the legitimacy of beliefs about the environment, but about how we could so much as have such beliefs at all. Much of the relevant section is taken up with his attempt to deal with the latter question. There is no need to go into that here. All the same it is worth noting that Hume's preoccupation with explaining why we have any beliefs about the environment, and his pessimism over how such beliefs could be legitimate, require no revision of the claim that he is a normative epistemologist. What is true is that Hume is faced with a major difficulty for his normative epistemology which he does not know how to solve. For our present purposes the interesting question to consider is whether there are lessons to be learnt from Hume's difficulties.

A large part of the problem stems from the fact that Hume regards experiences as objects of perception. This is no mere oversight on Hume's part for he argues the point. As it concerns sensory experiences, or impressions, the argument is that since (*a*) perception presents us with impressions but (*b*) perception does not present us with a double existence, impressions plus something else, (*c*) impressions are the only objects of perception. The mistake in the argument has to do with the interpretation of (*a*). Perception does present us with impressions. This just means that through perception we have impressions. It does not mean that impressions are what we perceive, but this is just what Hume reads into (*a*).[13]

[13] Unfortunately, as I implied in the Introduction, philosophers still find difficulties in the very idea of there being experiences conceived as conscious occurrences, not reducible to inclinations or the onset of inclinations to belief, on the grounds that we directly perceive things in the world around us. There are suggestions of such a line of thought in Heil (1983), p. 75. Pitcher (1971) is mainly concerned to attack sense-datum theories but there are hints on pp. 39 ff. of the view that we do not have sensations because if we had they would be objects of awareness. It is certainly true that we do not perceive things via the perception or awareness of experiences, sensations, or whatever. The view defended in this book does not imply otherwise.

The upshot is the mistaken view that the inference habits we acquire through experience take us from beliefs about experiences to beliefs about experiences. Accordingly, Hume thinks that

> as long as we take our perceptions and objects to be the same, we can never infer the existence of the one from that of the other, nor form any argument from the relation of cause and effect. (I. iv. ii. 193)

One might be tempted to suppose that the difficulties Hume encounters in this area would vanish once the mistaken view that experiences are objects of perception is abandoned. For then there might seem to be a prospect of treating *E*-beliefs in a manner which is rather similar to Hume's treatment of generalization. In discussing generalization Hume is at pains to point out that there are no reasons for opting into the practice of making generalizations from observations. Nor do we need such reasons since we are generalizers by nature. Nevertheless, he thinks that some ways of arriving at generalizations are better than others. In particular, he thinks it is important to take account of the possibility that we may be influenced by 'accidental circumstances'. The parallel in the case of *E*-beliefs would be this. There are no reasons for opting into the practice of basing beliefs about the present environment on current experience. Nor do we need such reasons since we are naturally constituted so as to form beliefs in this way. Nevertheless, there are ways of forming such beliefs which are better than others. In particular, we need to take into account the possibility that in some circumstances there will be relevant countervailing facts.

For Hume the matter would not be quite so straightforward, however. Not, at any rate, if he were to accept that *F*-type experiences contribute to the justification of beliefs to the effect that something having the look of an *F* is before one only given the assumption that in general the occurrence of such experiences is strong fallible evidence of the presence of such things. The problem is that within Hume's framework all evidential links are contingent. The evidential link in question would obtain only if it were true as a matter of fact that usually when *F*-type experiences occur something having the look of an *F* is before the subject. To be acceptable such a generalization would have to be confirmed by perceived conjunctions of *F*-type experiences and the presence of things having the look of *F*s. But such confirmation is impossible since such conjunctions are 'never present to the mind'. To avoid Hume's difficulties we must not only abandon the idea that experiences are objects, we must also show that justified experience-based beliefs are not justificationally dependent on empirically grounded beliefs in generalizations connecting the occurrence of experiences with the presence of objects. According to the account given in Chapter 4 this last requirement is satisfied via the idea that possessing the concept of something having the look of an *F* commits you to thinking of the occurrence of *F*-type experiences as strong fallible evidence that an *F* is there. Within Hume's framework there is no room for such an idea.

It is even clearer in the case of *E*-beliefs than it is in the case of ordinary empirical generalizations that such understanding as we have of the relevant justificational constraints does not derive from a Humean review of the operations of the understanding. If we can reach some understanding of what goes on when we arrive at a belief about the present environment in the usual unstudied way in response to current experience, it is because we already know what the relevant constraints are. We arrive at this knowledge by becoming explicitly aware of the sorts of considerations to which we appeal in evaluating *E*-beliefs and the sorts of considerations which we take into account in forming and maintaining *E*-beliefs. But that is at least in part a matter of coming to a perspicuous view of our conceptual capacities by self-consciously exercising them in relation to actual or imagined examples. It is not an enquiry into the aetiology of past judgements.

The kind of activity whereby we become aware of the nature of our conceptual capacities could itself be conceived as an enquiry into the operations of the understanding. Some readers may feel that a more charitable reading of Hume and Locke would take them to be engaged in just such an exercise. I think what can be said is that the insights which both Locke and Hume have about the ways in which we form beliefs spring from what is in fact reflection on acquired conceptual capacities of various types. But each takes himself to be penetrating beyond these to the native capacities responsible for belief and concept acquisition. This is understandable because, as I have stressed already, a conception of the justificational constraints relevant to some class of beliefs has implications for how in practice such beliefs can be acquired and maintained. The real thrust of my criticism of both Locke and Hume is that they misconceive the order of enquiry as between basic cognitive capacities and acquired conceptual capacities. Locke is led to do so because he thinks that we can scrutinize experience for indications of the concepts which are available to us. Hume is led to do so by his eagerness to apply the experimental method to the mind. Both fail to see that such models as we are able to frame about basic cognitive capacities depend on our understanding of conceptual capacities.

5.4. *Naturalized Epistemology*

Although 'human knowledge, its scope and limits' is not on the philosophical agenda in the way that it was, there is a growing tendency among philosophers to assume that the methods of natural science, whatever precisely they may be, are definitive of serious systematic enquiry. W. V. Quine has been immensely influential in this respect. Like Hume and Locke, his view of what constitutes reasonable enquiry is much influenced by prior assumptions about our cognitive capacities and especially by two 'cardinal tenets of empiricism'[14] which he regards as unassailable. These are, firstly, that 'whatever evidence there *is* for science *is* sensory evidence' and, secondly, that 'all inculcation of meanings of words must rest ultimately on sensory evidence' (*EN*, p. 75). Quine is a revisionary nativist of the old school. On the basis of an understanding of our cognitive capacities he seeks to curb profligate theorizing, especially in the fields of psychology and linguistics. That is the whole thrust of his detailed work on meaning and the mental, and is at least part of the motivation of his concern with the nature of a regimented language for science which would be capable of expressing 'all traits of reality worthy of the name' (*WO*, p. 228).[15]

[14] See Quine (1969*a*) in Quine (1969*b*) and Kornblith (1985). Page references in the text are to Quine (1969*b*) and are prefixed by '*EN*'.

[15] Quine (1960). Page references in the text are prefixed by '*WO*'.

Quine himself stresses the discontinuities between his own work and that of earlier philosophers. One in particular is central to his conception of epistemology. Traditional epistemologists, on Quine's reading, sought to legitimize science by ensuring that it could be built on proper evidential foundations. Their aim, he thinks, was an epistemology which would 'contain . . . natural science' by constructing it from sense data (*EN*, p. 83). This meant that they could not without circularity use natural science in providing an account of how science is constructed. Quine's aim, by contrast, is an epistemology which is 'contained in natural science, as a chapter of psychology' (*EN*, p. 83), a naturalized epistemology, conceived as a scientific enterprise like any other with its subject-matter, cognition, conceived as a natural phenomenon like any other. Conducted in this spirit epistemology would use the best of current science to study 'how the human subject of our study posits bodies and projects his physics from his data' (*EN*, p. 83). On this view of the matter there is no circularity problem

> once we have stopped dreaming of deducing science from observations. If we are out simply to understand the link between observation and science, we are well advised to use any available information, including that provided by the very science whose link with observation we are seeking to understand. (*EN*, p. 76)

What are we to make of this? It is actually quite difficult to find epistemologists who, like Descartes, have adopted the standpoint of solitary enquirers trying to find a reason to venture beyond the contents of consciousness without relying on science or common sense, and who have regarded this project as a step on the way to legitimizing science and common sense. Bertrand Russell's *Our Knowledge of the External World*[16] shows the influence of Descartes, yet in that work Russell warns his readers that '[t]here is not any superfine brand of knowledge, obtainable by the philosopher, which can give us a standpoint from which to criticize the whole of the knowledge of daily life'.[17] Whatever may be said of others it is clear enough that neither Locke nor Hume took up Descartes' project. Locke's 'historical, plain method' (I. i. 1) and Hume's 'experimental

[16] Russell (1926).
[17] Ibid., p. 73.

method' take reasonable enquiry to be a going concern and are happy to rely upon common-sense judgements in their deliberations. Locke is dismissive of Descartes' scepticism (IV. ii. 14) and Hume deliberately distances himself from the Cartesian project when he stresses the pointlessness of trying to legitimize by argument our 'faculty' for generalizing from past experience.

Both Locke and Hume saw themselves as revisionists. Backed up by an improved understanding of our cognitive capacities they wished to place an embargo on certain types of enquiry and recommend sound procedures for others. In this respect they are no different from Quine. If they do not draw upon natural science it is because the natural science of the day had little if anything to say about our cognitive capacities; not because of a worry about the circularity involved in using science to legitimize science.

It might be argued that there is a matter on which Quine is significantly at odds with traditional epistemologists. If epistemology is a chapter of psychology, if its aim is to 'understand the link between science and observation', then it might seem to be solely concerned with how we acquire the beliefs we do. Since traditional epistemology is a normative discipline concerned with constraints on justified belief, Quine's naturalized epistemology might seem to involve a radical departure from tradition.

The trouble with this line of thought is that assumptions about the constraints on justified belief are crucially important for Quine's critical endeavours. These assumptions determine the sorts of data which Quine regards as relevant to, for example, the scientific study of language use. If Quine is right then in this area we have to rely only on observable behaviour, narrowly conceived, plus some loose maxims enjoining us to plump for the simplest theories which least disturb entrenched theory. It turns out that beliefs, hopes, wishes, intentions, and propositional attitudes generally become suspect because ascriptions of attitudes are highly underdetermined by the available data and the maxims. Indeed, the very concepts we have of the attitudes are shaky because they resist explication in terms of behaviour. Quine infers that there is no proper science of beliefs and other such mental states, or, at least, none which occupies itself with these states *qua* propositional attitudes (*WO*, pp. 216–21).[18] And 'no proper science' means no knowledge worthy of the name.

I mention this conception of the psychology of language-use only to illustrate my earlier contention that Quine is indeed a normative epistemologist and as such must rely on a conception of the constraints on justified belief. If epistemology is to become a chapter of psychology, psychology is going to have to include some consideration of these constraints. Be that as it may we need to focus now on the question of whether, and if so how, naturalized epistemology can vindicate some particular view of what the constraints are. This has a crucial bearing on the wider question of how the study of basic cognitive capacities bears on the normative concerns of epistemology.

Quine neatly summarizes the basic presuppositions of his naturalized epistemology in the following passage.[19]

> Science tells us that our only source of information about the external world is through the impact of light rays and molecules upon our sensory surfaces. Stimulated in these ways we somehow evolve an elaborate and useful science. (*NNK*, p. 68)

A developed scientific epistemology would explain how we get from stimulation to a complex web of belief. Quine himself contributes to this project through a study of how language might have been acquired. To the uninitiated the emphasis on language might seem not to be to the point. The underlying rationale derives from a central tenet of Quine's general theory of language to the effect that there is no clear distinction to be made between language, on the one hand, and theory or belief

[18] I do not wish to imply that Quine's criticism of mentalistic or 'folk' psychology is entirely epistemological in character. As Hookway points out (1988), p. 137, Quine is guided by the idea 'that the only physical facts which could possibly be relevant to fixing the correctness of translation manuals [and thus of attributions of propositional attitudes] are facts about stimulus meanings', which is to say, facts about behavioural dispositions. He is also influenced by the idea that the logic of statements ascribing propositional attitudes is irredeemably obscure. I am inclined to think, nevertheless, that while neither of these ideas is itself epistemological the attractiveness to Quine of at least the former lies in the fact that it meshes with the hard-nosed empiricism which he thinks is warranted by the scientific study of 'the evidential link'. See below.

[19] See Quine (1975) in Guttenplan (1975). Page references are prefixed by '*NNK*'.

on the other, nor therefore between language learning and the acquisition of belief or theory. Indeed, Quine thinks that the 'evidential relation', that is, the relation between belief and evidence, is 'virtually enacted . . . in the learning', holding out the prospect that a study of language acquisition will furnish clues 'for the scientific study of scientific method and evidence' (*NNK*, pp. 74–5).

We have already had occasion (4.1) to note that Quine has no place for a concept of experience of the sort developed in this book. He deals in sensory stimulations conceived as irradiations of nerve-endings. At the core of his discussion of evidence is the idea that stimulations of certain types dispose the subject to assent to sentences of certain types. In explaining this idea more fully I shall do so in a way which facilitates comparison with the view of the justificatory role of experience which was presented in Chapter 4. I shall help myself to some concepts and terminology which Quine does not himself use.

The linchpin of Quine's epistemology is the notion of an observation sentence. An observation sentence is one which satisfies the condition that 'all speakers of the language give the same verdict [assent or dissent, as the case may be] when given the same concurrent stimulation' (*EN*, pp. 867). Thus the sentence 'There is a red thing there' would be an observation sentence but 'There is a bank manager there' would not be.[20] Those who know that John is a bank manager may be disposed by the visual stimulations they receive when they look at him to assent to the latter sentence. Others who do not know John would be likely not to assent or dissent under the very same stimulations. Since verdicts to the sentence vary under the same stimulations the sentence is not an observation sentence.

We can sharpen up the discussion by introducing a variant of the *F*-type typology (1.4). Thus, an *F*-type stimulation is, roughly speaking, a stimulation of a type which an *F* would yield. An *F*-indicating stimulation would be one of a type occurrences of which reliably indicate the presence of an *F*. The occurrence of an *F*-indicating stimulation is strong fallible evidence of the presence of an *F* in the sense explained in 2.4.

[20] This assumes a liberal conception of observationality. Quine allows that observationality admits of degrees. The example given is at least nearer to the purest observationality than that with which it is contrasted.

Yet *F*-indicating stimulations do not usually constitute evidence that is available to the subject for experience-based applications of the concept of an *F*, since the subject usually has no idea of what is happening at his nerve-endings. This raises a problem about how the 'evidential relation' connects with the constraints on justified experience-based beliefs. How are we to make sense of the idea that a belief about the present scene is justifiably based on current stimulation?

The problem here has nothing to do with the project of using epistemology to legitimize science. Nor, more specifically, has it anything to do with a worry about how a solitary enquirer who suspends belief about the external world could come to have reason to believe anything at all about that world. The problem is simply that any adequate epistemology must give an account of the conditions of justified belief. That stimulations can have evidential links with beliefs does not of itself supply such an account.

According to the conception of justification presented in previous chapters a belief derives justification, at least in part, from a state only if there is an appropriate rational connection between the state, or some complex of which the state is a part, and the belief. It is a consequence of our Competence conditions (2.2, 4.3) that the subject of the belief must have a conception of what counts as a rational connection and be capable of evaluating beliefs with respect to justification in the light of whether an appropriate rational connection obtains. This being so the state in question must be of a sort by reference to which beliefs are routinely evaluated for justification both by the subjects of these beliefs and by others. I argued in Chapter 4 that sensory experiences, as I conceive them, meet this condition. Stimulations do not since they are not routinely available either to the subjects of beliefs or to others. Indeed, the very idea that we have stimulations, conceived as irradiations of nerve-endings, could be dropped without any loss to our ability to evaluate beliefs which are not about stimulations. There are two ways of arguing that this does not matter. One is to hold that there is no need to worry about how stimulations could contribute to the justification of beliefs on the grounds that justification is solely concerned with beliefs and relations between beliefs. This is the line which Davidson takes in the paper cited earlier (4.1). It is at odds with the aims of Quine's study of the 'evidential relation'. Quine cannot be content with the idea that the relation between stimulations and beliefs is merely causal. He thinks our beliefs ought to be rigorously controlled by the evidence of the senses.

Another way of defusing the problem is to follow Goldman in adopting a non-regulative account of justification (4.7). Goldman is sensitive, in a way that Quine is not, to the problems of giving an account of the norms or standards of justified belief as opposed to describing cognitive processes. He makes quite explicit the sort of relation between processes and justification to which, as I have argued (5.3), Hume was feeling his way. Leaving aside refinements, Goldman thinks that a belief is justified if and only if it is permitted by a right system of justificational rules.[21] A right system of rules is one which permits reliable processes of belief acquisition. More precisely, a system of rules *R* is right if and only if

> *R* permits certain (basic) psychological processes [i.e. ones which are native, not acquired], and the instantiation of these processes would result in a truth ratio of beliefs [i.e. a ratio of true over total beliefs] that meets some specified high threshold (greater than ·50).[22]

Note that this condition of rule rightness may be satisfied by systems of non-regulative rules. That is why the general approach is congenial to Quine's type of epistemology. An example of a reliable process would be acquiring the belief that a red thing is before you when you have (red thing)-type stimulations. Rules permitting the acquisition of beliefs of certain types on the occurrence of stimulations of certain corresponding types could not be rules which guide, for essentially the reasons mentioned already. But if Goldman is right they could be non-regulative rules suitable for appraising stimulation-based beliefs.

The question then is whether Quine's revisionary nativism, fleshed out with a Goldman-type account of justification, is satisfactory. I think it is not for the following reasons.

Obviously, it would beg the question to argue that since conceptualism (5.1) is true any non-regulative account of justification must be wrong. On the other hand, conceptualism is attractive because, among other things, it seems to capture the

[21] See Goldman (1986), pp. 59 ff.
[22] Ibid., p. 106.

requirements which we acknowledge in practice when we evaluate beliefs with respect to justification. So, at the very least, it should trouble Quine and Goldman that there is a plausible theory of justification which has a central role for the idea that we are governed by inference and quasi-inference patterns and copes with difficult cases like *E*-beliefs. It is worth recalling that Goldman rejects regulative conceptions of justification on the assumption that regulative norms would guide in the way that sets of instructions guide. But as we noted in 4.5 this does not take account of a far more plausible alternative.

Another problem arises from the fact that Quine's account of the 'evidential relation' does not take account of the full range of considerations which can be invoked when beliefs are evaluated with respect to justification. In particular, it does not take into account first-person evaluations of *E*-beliefs involving the replay of sensory experiences as described in 4.2. This constitutes an objection to the attempt to understand belief acquisition in terms of stimulations rather than experiences considered as conscious occurrences. What enables us to put this objection is the fact that our actual practice shows that we make the kind of evaluations mentioned. We need detailed models of the conceptual practices which are involved in belief evaluation if we are to understand the processes of belief acquisition. No one could reasonably deny that stimulations are implicated in the production of beliefs, but which beliefs we extract from the stimulations we receive depends on acquired conceptual capacities. Quine does not suggest otherwise, though he would express the point in terms of acquired dispositions to give verdicts to sentences. But, like Locke and Hume, he reverses the proper order of enquiry in epistemology. To cast light on the processes involved in acquiring beliefs we must have an understanding of our conceptual capacities. The scientific study of the route from stimulations to beliefs will not itself yield such an understanding. This is not to deny that much of what Quine tells us about belief acquisition is relevant to epistemology. It is relevant because it illuminates the psychology of basing beliefs. But it achieves that illumination to the extent that the psychology plausibly reflects the pattern-governed ways in which we form, maintain, and evaluate beliefs. These ways may lead us to the underlying basic processes but we should not expect the processes to tell us how to go about acquiring beliefs.

The role of conceptual capacities in acquiring beliefs raises problems for a distinction which is fundamental to Goldman's conception of epistemology. Goldman distinguishes between basic psychological processes and acquired methods, such as algorithms, heuristics, skills, and techniques. The former fall within the scope of what he calls primary epistemology, while the latter are the concern of secondary epistemology. Goldman thinks that it is possible to distinguish between two corresponding levels of justification: primary justifiedness and secondary justifiedness. The former results from the use of basic processes and the latter from the use of acquired and approved methods. He also seems to think that we can do primary epistemology without venturing much into secondary epistemology.[23] The difficulties I have with this should come as no surprise against the background of the previous discussion. Perception is a basic process and various aspects of perception can be studied with little if any regard to what Goldman would count as acquired methods. But perception is of interest to epistemology in so far as it is a means whereby beliefs are acquired. So as epistemologists we have to consider how sensory experiences interact with conceptual capacities. Since conceptual capacities presumably fall under the heading of acquired methods, epistemologically relevant studies of perception cannot proceed solely at the level of Goldman's primary epistemology. More importantly, it is difficult to see how, in view of the essential role of conceptual capacities, and thus acquired methods, in belief acquisition, we can make any sense of the distinction between primary and secondary justifiedness. When a belief is justified certain native capacities will have been at work implementing, among other things, the relevant conceptual capacities. But there is no way of isolating a level of justification which is due to native capacities from a level which is due to acquired methods.

There are other difficulties concerning the feasibility of reliabilist accounts of justification which have received extensive discussion in the literature.[24] I have confined myself to criticisms of Quine and Goldman which serve to reinforce the central negative theme of the present chapter. Nativism is not a plausible alternative to conceptualism.

[23] See Goldman (1986), p. 93.

[24] For detailed criticisms of reliability theories of justified belief, see Bonjour (1985) and Luper-Foy (1985).

6

Groundless Beliefs

6.1. *Foundationalism*

Chapter 2 presented a number of conditions which have to be fulfilled if a belief that *p* is to derive its justification from beliefs that *q*, that *r*, ... One of these conditions was the Basis condition *JUS4* which required that the contents of the basis beliefs that *q*, that *r*, . . . be legitimately taken for granted. In Chapter 4 a somewhat similar condition was introduced for cases in which a belief derives its justification in part from current experience and in part from another belief. This condition also requires that the content of the basis belief be legitimately taken for granted. Thus far I have recognized that we may legitimately take for granted propositions which we are derivatively justified in believing and propositions which are normative. I shall have a good deal more to say about normative propositions later in this chapter. To begin with I shall take up the question of whether, and if so how, derived justification comes to an end. If any basis beliefs are themselves derivatively justified then they in turn derive their justification from other beliefs, and so on. The picture which this suggests is that there are branching chains of derived justification as in Figure 2 in which justification is transmitted upwards. The beliefs which occur at the nodes are believings of some particular individual.

It seems natural to conceive of derived justification as being transitive. If the belief that *p* derives its justification from the beliefs that *q*, and that *r*, and if each of these beliefs derives its justification in the manner represented in Figure 2, then the belief that *p* derives its justification from the beliefs that *s*, that *t*, that *u*, that *v*, and that *w*. A belief may be said to be justificationally dependent on any belief which is an element in any set of beliefs from which it derives its justification. In the

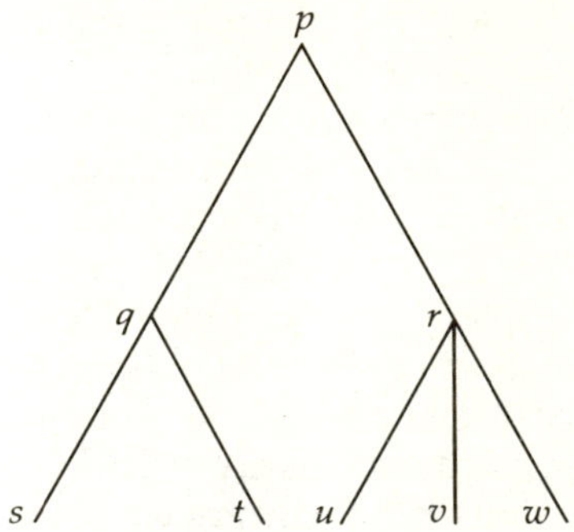

FIG. 2

system represented in the diagram the belief that *p* is justificationally dependent on all the beliefs which occur below it. The question to consider is whether the branches of chains of justification must terminate and, if so, what kind of beliefs can occupy the termini. I am assuming here that the branches are concerned solely with beliefs, but obviously the situation is complicated if beliefs can be justificationally dependent on experiences as argued in Chapter 4. Leaving that complication aside for a moment let us focus on beliefs.

It is arguable that the branches of chains of derived justification must terminate. Suppose that they do not. It seems then that their branches must be linear and infinitely long, or circular. A branch is linear provided that no belief in it is justificationally dependent on any belief which is justificationally dependent on it. A branch is circular if it is not linear. There are objections to each of the alternatives mentioned. One objection to the first is that finite individuals cannot have infinitely many beliefs and so no branch could be infinitely long. Another which is close to the central concerns of the present work assumes a regulative conception of justification. According to such a conception it must be possible for a subject to recapitulate the chains through which his beliefs derive their justification. If a belief *B* is justificationally dependent on a belief *B*' then the subject must hold *B* under the guidance of the relevant inference patterns. But being thus guided requires one to have the capacity to take *B*' into account as a component in the causal ancestry of *B*. But if *B*' is out of reach, because infinitely far along the branch, no such recapitulation would be possible.

There is a powerful objection to the second alternative along the following lines. If a belief *B* is justificationally dependent on a belief *B*' then *B* must be causally dependent on *B*' in the sense that the subject has *B* at least in part because he has *B*'. Circular branching would require there to be beliefs which are, in the relevant sense, causally dependent on beliefs which are causally dependent on them, and that is not possible.

If the foregoing considerations are sound then the branches of chains of justification must terminate. One view about the structure of justification which incorporates a distinctive view of how the branches terminate is *foundationalism*. Though I reject foundationalism it is of some importance to see why it will not do.

To formulate foundationalism we need first of all a classification of a subject's beliefs into *basic* and *non-basic*. Your belief that *p* is basic if it is not based on any other beliefs and non-basic if it is based on some other beliefs. Stated in this way the distinction is not especially interesting or problematic. It allows for the possibility that a belief may be basic for a person at one time but non-basic for that person at another time, or for another person at the same or a different time. For example, if you now believe that Stirling has a castle because you think someone is telling you that Stirling has a castle, your belief is non-basic. But if the same belief has long been part of the stored background of beliefs you carry around with you then it might well be basic, for it may not be causally dependent, in the sense just explained, on any other beliefs. You may well have come to believe it because of some other beliefs, but it may not now be based on any other beliefs.

In this connection it is important not to infer from the claim that a belief is basic that other beliefs are irrelevant to your holding it. If you ceased to believe that there is a town called Stirling you would cease to believe that Stirling has a castle. To say that the latter belief is basic is to say only that there is no set of beliefs such that you have the given belief because you have the beliefs in the set. You do not believe that Stirling has a castle because you believe that Stirling has a town and there need be no set of beliefs such that you believe that Stirling has a castle because you have the beliefs in the set. Some beliefs can just be stored without being sustained by other beliefs.

Two other matters deserve particular attention. One is that the distinction between basic and non-basic does not concern whether the beliefs in question are legitimate. Basic and non-basic beliefs may or may not be legitimate. The other is that the distinction does not turn on a distinction between types of belief content, but rather on the causal role of beliefs within the network of a subject's beliefs at a given time. This is illustrated by the example just mentioned where beliefs with the same content might be basic within one person's network of beliefs but not within another person's network of beliefs.[1]

The distinction between basic and non-basic beliefs does not yet give us foundationalism. Foundationalism worthy of the name involves at least the following further claims: first, that only beliefs with a certain type of content can be properly or legitimately basic,[2] secondly, that legitimately held non-basic beliefs must be justified, and thirdly, that for any justified non-basic belief there is a set of properly basic beliefs from which it derives its justification. (It should be recalled that I reserve the term 'justified belief' for derivatively justified beliefs. The notion of a legitimate belief covers both justified beliefs and, on my view, also certain groundless beliefs.) Let us focus on the foundations of beliefs about the world, leaving aside mathematical, logical, and conceptual matters. What sorts of propositions are suitable to be contents of properly basic beliefs serving as foundations for beliefs about the world?

One line of thought is that if the belief that *p* is properly basic then it must be that the subject of the belief cannot be mistaken in believing that *p*.[3] One might be tempted to suppose that a belief that a red thing is there, based on current experience, could not mistaken. But on reflection it is pretty clear that this is not so. The subject may have a (red thing)-type experience but fail to take account of relevant countervailing facts. It is not surprising that foundationalists have inclined towards the view that the only properly basic beliefs serving as foundations for

[1] Compare Kornblith (1980) in Kornblith (1985).

[2] The terminology and the concept of proper basicality is used in Plantinga (1982). This paper includes a penetrating critical examination of foundationalism.

[3] See Pollock (1987), pp. 27 ff., on this idea.

beliefs about the environment are beliefs about one's own current sensory or memory experience. The idea here is that we cannot be mistaken about the sorts of experiences we are having in the way that we can be mistaken about what is before us. While it is understandable that this should be thought to be so it is open to objection. If the relevant beliefs about current experience concern their type then there is reason to think that they can be mistaken. It is likely that our beliefs as to the types of our current experiences often depend on the beliefs, or at least dispositions to belief, which these experiences cause us to have. If you think that your current experience is (red thing)-type this may be because it is such that it seems to you that a red thing is before you, in the special sense of Chapters 1 and 4. But as I argued in 4.2 in connection with the nectarines example, experiences can be out of kilter with their contents. An experience which is not *F*-type can nevertheless be such that it seems to you that an *F* is there. It is perhaps not obvious that this could happen in the case of experiences such that it seems to you that a red thing is there. Yet it seems to be possible in principle. If a person has a habit of making over-hasty judgements about the colours of objects it could be that it seems to him that a red thing is there on occasions in which he has a (brown thing)-type experience. But then such a person might conceivably make over-hasty judgements about his visual experiences too, believing that they are (red thing)-type when they are not.

Even if the view of proper basicality which I have just criticized were granted it would remain an open question whether beliefs can be justificationally dependent on current experiences, as I argued in Chapter 4. If they can be then it has to be acknowledged that the branches of chains of justification can terminate in experiences rather than beliefs. In that case basic beliefs may be derivatively justified although they are not justificationally dependent on other beliefs. We could describe as *experiential* the sort of foundationalism which has it that the justification of all beliefs about the environment ultimately derives from experiences. *Doxastic* foundationalism, by contrast, has it that the justification of all such beliefs ultimately derives from properly basic beliefs, albeit beliefs about experiences.

In the present context the significance of foundationalism is that it rules out the possibility that the sorts of beliefs which on my view have normative propositions as contents are properly basic. Take, for instance, propositions to the effect that the occurrence of behaviour of certain kinds is strong fallible evidence that the subject is in pain. According to the account proposed in 3.2 these propositions have a normative role for us and may be legitimately taken for granted even in the absence of grounds in their favour. Yet they would not figure as the contents of properly basic beliefs on any standard foundationalist view. So it is of some importance for my project that there should be good reason to reject foundationalism. It is also important to make very clear that my own emphasis on the idea that experiences can contribute to the justification of beliefs is not motivated by foundationalist considerations.

Despite its curious seductiveness, foundationalism is wholly implausible when understood in conjunction with any account of derived justification which links justification with causal dependence in the manner explained. The issue here is independent of the criticism offered above of the foundationalist conception of proper basicality. To take just one example: You come to believe that someone wishes to see you on hearing a knock on your study door. Such a belief may be justified. Among the beliefs which might have a role in this situation is the belief that the occurrence of knocking sounds coming from the region of the door is strong fallible evidence that someone wants to see you. The foundationalist must suppose that if this latter belief is legitimate it is justified, and that if justified then there must be a set of properly basic beliefs from which it derives justification. On a causal view of derived justification that would mean that the beliefs in question must be causally dependent on beliefs about current sensory or memory experience. And if the experiential version of foundationalism is assumed the implication would be that the beliefs in question are causally dependent on current sensory or memory experiences themselves. But neither implication is realistic. There need be nothing about current sensory or memory experience which bears on the acquisition or maintenance of the beliefs in question.

This last point is so obvious that it might seem puzzling that foundationalism could ever have seemed attractive. Part of the reason why it has is that foundationalists have not always held that justificational dependence implies causal dependence. They have thought of the justification of a belief in terms of the considerations which the subject could advance in support of the proposition believed.[4] This approach may yield insights into justification because it demands examination of, among other things, the inferential structures involved in justification. But unless the grasp of an inferential structure has something to do with why one actually holds a belief, it is difficult to see how it can be relevant to the belief's being justified.

Even if the foundationalist were to make a good case for resisting the view that justificational dependence implies causal dependence, he would still have to face other problems, as we can see if we return to the example mentioned above. Consider what justificatory argument you might offer in support of the proposition that knocking sounds from the region of the door provide evidence that someone wants to see you. You might first of all point out that usually when knocking sounds of this sort occur and you say, 'Come in' or 'Open the door', it emerges that somebody wants to see you. To put the point more briefly, you rely on the generalization that, roughly speaking, knocking sounds herald someone wishing to see you. The foundationalist is going to have to claim that this latter generalization is supported by there having been a host of confirming instances and few, if any, disconfirming cases. But now a justificatory argument is needed to support the view that the empirical support did obtain. This might seem to present no difficulty. Probably you can think of many occasions on which the knocking sound heralded someone wishing to see you, and few occasions on which this was not so. The kind of foundationalist we are presently considering thinks that the ability to draw on stored memories in this way is what is important for the justification of the relevant generalization, not having current memory experiences.

This entire approach to the matter seems to me to be profoundly mistaken. For one thing it is conceivable that you might be unable to recall any specific occasions in which a knocking sound at the door heralds someone wishing to see

[4] Compare Kornblith's discussion of the argument-on-paper approach to justification, in Kornblith (1980).

you. It is far from clear that this should in any way cast doubt on your right to believe like everyone else the generalization that knocking sounds at the door herald people wishing to see you. You may be perfectly convinced that on countless occasions knocks on the door have been followed by people coming in wanting to see you, but this is compatible with your being unable to recall any specific occasion. This point leads naturally to another. It is true that if you were to test the generalization you would look for empirical support. But the foundationalist holds to the stronger thesis that to be justified in believing the generalization you have to be able to cite evidence in its support. You must therefore have an independent reason for thinking that the evidence obtains. This is where memory is supposed to come in. But why should it be thought that this way of thinking is correct? It assumes that the beliefs relating to evidence for the generalization are less vulnerable than belief in the generalization itself. Yet in practice you may be more confident about the truth of the generalization than you are about recollecting evidence in its support. An account of justification which reflects our evaluative practice could not with any plausibility forbid such relative confidence. The position is not improved by introducing testimony as a source of justification for beliefs. Testimony could only be relevant through being recalled and so again there would arise the question why we should have to be able to recall testimony in order for it to be legitimate to retain beliefs acquired by its means.

A psychologically realistic account of the matter must countenance legitimately held yet groundless beliefs. Included in this class would be your belief that the occurrence of knocking sounds coming from the region of one's office-door is strong fallible evidence that someone wants to see one. The content of this belief arguably has a normative role in our thinking in the sense explained in 3.2. We learn to count it true as we learn the practice of telling that someone wants to see us from knocks on our doors. Repeated instances of knocking sounds heralding someone wishing to see us may have had a role in inculcating the practice, but if the foregoing discussion is correct we should be wary of concluding that our present belief in the evidential link in question is based on, and derives justification from, beliefs to the effect that such instances have obtained.

It is time now to say more about normative propositions and to take a look in particular at Wittgenstein's remarks in *On Certainty*. Wittgenstein appears to contemplate the possibility that a very wide range of propositions have a normative status.

6.2. *Wittgenstein and Normativity*

In 'A Defence of Common Sense'[5] G. E. Moore listed various things which he said he knew, such as that there is a body which is his and which was born at a certain time in the past, had existed continuously ever since, had always been in contact with or close to the earth, in an environment containing three-dimensional objects, including large numbers of other human bodies; that the earth had existed long before he was born, and contained human beings who had died long before he was born; that he and other human beings had had various experiences and observed various facts to obtain in the environment, and so forth. Moore also said that he knew that others knew such things with respect to themselves. Wittgenstein thinks there is something odd about saying you know such things and in *On Certainty*[6] he tries to pin down the source of the sense of oddity.

The remarks in *On Certainty* are exploratory and unsystematic, so there is a considerable risk that any attempt at concise exposition will over-simplify or distort. Nevertheless, it seems fairly clear that there are two principal assumptions underlying Wittgenstein's unease about Moore's claim to know the various truisms to be true. One is that you know that *p* only if you have adequate grounds for believing that *p* (18, 91, 438 ff.). The other is that you know that *p* only if the proposition that *p* is one with respect to which the possibility of doubt is not ruled out (117; cf. 58, 121). Though it is difficult to find straightforward statements in the text, much of the discussion is germane to Moore only if some such assumptions are being made. The view seems to be that Moore's truisms are not the sorts of things one can appropriately say one knows to be true, in a sense of 'know' in which the two assumptions are true. For although each of us

[5] Moore (1959).

[6] References in the text are to the numbered paragraphs of Wittgenstein (1969).

accepts truisms corresponding to those Moore said he knew, we have no grounds for believing them true and they are the sorts of propositions with respect to which, in Wittgenstein's view, the possibility of doubt is ruled out in the usual contexts in which such propositions may figure. So some special stage setting would be necessary to make sense of Moore's claims to knowledge and Moore does not provide it.

I shall set aside the issue about the appropriate use of the verb 'to know' and concentrate on the considerations about grounds and about doubt. Much of the discussion in *On Certainty* is concerned with trying to make it plausible that groundless believing is sometimes legitimate even where the propositions in question are not self-evidently true in the usual sense. To this end Wittgenstein feels his way towards a view of the special status of certain kinds of propositions and of beliefs to the effect that they are true.

A key theme is that there are propositions which have 'the form of empirical propositions' (96) and yet their 'role is like that of rules of a game' (95). Together they form a system or world-picture, but this 'is not a more or less arbitrary point of departure for all our arguments'. On the contrary 'it belongs to the essence of what we call an argument'. It is 'the element in which arguments have their life' (105). Wittgenstein appears to treat the following as examples of propositions of this type.

> Mountains exist for a very long time. (143)
>
> Things do not vanish or cease to exist when you stop looking at them. (153, 163)
>
> If a substance acts in a certain way in certain circumstances it will act in the same way in relevantly similar circumstances. (167 ff.)
>
> Modern maps are pretty accurate. (170)
>
> Scientific textbooks can be trusted. (600)

It is not very clear what Wittgenstein means by saying that these propositions have the form of empirical propositions. Presumably he wishes to imply at least that they are not logical or conceptual truths on any received view, and also that, on the face of it, they are the sorts of propositions which on standard empiricist theories would not be acceptable unless on the basis of evidence (401). The principal claim, however, is that such propositions can have a role which is like that of the rules of a game. The claim is, I take it, that they have a normative role. Wittgenstein does not spell out what this means, but what he says seems to be consistent with the considerations about normative propositions introduced in 3.2. Crucially, they are propositions which govern our thinking in such a way that they are placed beyond doubt and dispute and the need for support.[7]

Wittgenstein says that propositions of this kind make up the inherited background against which people distinguish between true and false. People who more or less tacitly rely on them do not do so because they have satisfied themselves of their correctness. Rather they have come to share the perspective into which these propositions enter in something like the way in which they have acquired language. In both cases it is a matter of acquiring skills by a combination of explicit teaching and immersion in a context in which the skills are exercised. So, for example, although you may never have thought to yourself that mountains exist for a very long time or that modern maps are by and large accurate, the way you reason and the things you do may express a tacit commitment to these truths. If you want to know where exactly Madrid is you look it up in an atlas. If you are wondering what sort of creatures inhabited your area in Roman times you don't bother about whether the mountains in the area were there at that time. You show your tacit belief that they were through your considering only birds and animals which inhabit mountain regions.

What is the relation between these normative propositions and Moore's truisms? Wittgenstein is not explicit on this matter and yet it is not straightforward. Presumably, if normative propositions are to form part of an 'inherited background' they must be accepted by everyone for whom they are normative. In that case they cannot be specifically about, for instance, individuals who might not be known to all who are in the

[7] A conception of normativity in some respects akin to that employed here figures prominently in Crispin Wright's interpretation of Wittgenstein's philosophy of mathematics. See Wright (1980), esp. chs. 17 and 21. Wright's principal concern is with whether such a conception can plausibly explicate the notion of necessity. However, he notes on p. 413 that any such account is problematic since it is liable to let in statements which we should not ordinarily reckon as necessary.

relevant group. Many of Moore's truisms, however, are specifically about Moore. They concern his body, his environment, the time prior to his birth, and so on. They are also self-referring in that they are propositions which would be expressed by Moore's uttering certain sentences containing the first-person pronoun 'I'. So they are not just about Moore, they are propositions which articulate thoughts which Moore has about himself. On the face of it, then, the truisms should not count as normative propositions and yet Wittgenstein seems to slide indifferently from remarks about them, or parallel truisms concerning himself, to remarks about propositions, such as those listed above, which could plausibly be regarded as forming part of an inherited background. Nevertheless, corresponding to each of Moore's truisms and the parallels concerning ourselves, there is a more general proposition of which the truisms are a consequence. An example would be that each of us was born at a certain time and has existed continuously ever since. I shall concentrate on propositions in this latter class, together with those which are akin to the ones listed above, since these seem more suited to the role of normative proposition. It is interesting to note in passing that if, as seems likely, we base our acceptance of truisms like Moore's on our acceptance of the corresponding more general propositions, then there is a sense in which our acceptance of the truisms is not groundless. This would not, I think, undermine the main thrust of Wittgenstein's discussion. He is concerned with the kind of grounds which are supposed to be more certain than what they are grounds for, and the beliefs on which beliefs in the truisms are based need be no more certain than beliefs in the truisms.

There is a delicate matter which needs to be tackled before we can proceed. It seems to me to be natural to conceive of the normativity of propositions in such a way that one and the same proposition may be normative in one context and not in another. The notion of context is vague, to say the least. Following a convention adopted in 3.2, let us say that a *perspective* is a set of concepts and propositions. A group of people share a perspective if the members of the group share its constituent concepts and its constituent propositions are normative for that group. I do not think we go far wrong if we think of contexts as groups whose members share a perspective. Suppose now that propositions are individuated via their inferential and quasi-inferential powers, as determined by their conceptual and referential ingredients, and that the normativity of a proposition for a group is a function of its governing role for that group. Then there seems to be no reason why the same proposition could not be normative for a group which shares perspective *V*, yet not normative for a group which does not share *V*.

There are passages in which Wittgenstein could be read as endorsing this way of understanding normativity. He notes, for instance, that 'the same proposition may get treated at one time as something to test by experience, at another as a rule of testing' (98). However, we must treat such passages with caution. The German term which is translated as 'proposition' is 'Satz'. Although 'Satz' can mean proposition or thesis it can also mean sentence or phrase. The passage just quoted would not positively support the attribution to Wittgenstein of the proposed conception of normativity if 'Satz' were read as sentence. For that one and the same sentence could have a normative role in one context and not in another is consistent with the possibility that the sentence has different meanings in these different contexts and thus does not express the same proposition. I shall not pursue the exegetical issue. Whatever in detail Wittgenstein may have thought there is good reason to hold to the proposed conception of normativity and allow for the possibility that a proposition can be normative in one context and not in another.

If a proposition is normative for a group it is treated by the group as being indisputable. This does not mean that if people think a proposition is normative they treat it as being indisputable. In general people do not think of propositions as being normative or otherwise. It means that the normative propositions are ones which, among other things, people treat as being indisputable. Their being treated in this way is part of what it is for them to be normative. Doubt in relation to such propositions is ruled out, as Wittgenstein says. But many of the examples which Wittgenstein considers are not ones with respect to which it would be plausible to suppose that doubt is ruled out absolutely. It is possible to imagine contexts in which doubt, and with it dispute, could naturally and sensibly arise. This presents no problem for the proposed conception of normativity since according to that conception there need be nothing intrinsic to the propositions themselves, nothing about the propositions *qua* contents, which rules out doubt on the part of those who grasp them. Thus they need not be intrinsically self-evident in the way that the proposition that a triangle has three sides has been alleged to be. If this is right then we should not think of groups for whom certain propositions are normative as being forever bound by their normativity. Such groups would look askance at doubts about the propositions in question which were not backed up by any reasons for doubt, a point which Wittgenstein repeatedly stresses. But this is not to say that there could not be, or that the groups could not recognize, grounds for doubting some of the propositions which are normative for them.

This picture, of course, depends for its intelligibility on the legitimacy of distinguishing between what individuates a proposition and what makes the proposition normative for a group. But the legitimacy of such a distinction is guaranteed if propositions are individuated via their inferential and quasi-inferential powers and the normativity of a proposition consists in the fact that it governs our thinking in the sense previously explained. Some might wish to argue that the factors which make a proposition normative contribute to its individuation and on that basis reject the idea that a proposition can be normative in one context and not in another. Well, so they might, but they would need a theoretical framework at least as cogent as that presented here. No such framework is available and the best current work on the theory of content does not encourage optimism about attempts in that direction.

Somewhat similar issues arise in connection with the idea that normative propositions do not stand in need of support. If this is correct then beliefs with such propositions as contents, held by those for whom the propositions are normative, would not be open to censure even though neither derivatively justified nor properly basic on any foundationalist epistemology. Still, this is consistent with the possibility that there are contexts in which one would be open to censure for holding beliefs to the effect that such propositions are true unless one had grounds for thinking them true. *Whether not lacking grounds is a defect depends not just on the proposition believed but on its role in the context.* Again, the distinction between what individuates a proposition and what makes a proposition normative is crucial.

I have suggested that certain sorts of evidential propositions are normative. If Wittgenstein is right then the range of propositions which are normative for us is very wide indeed. Thus along with propositions which seem to be unavoidable presuppositions of any kind of systematic enquiry into nature, such as, that if a substance acts in a certain way in certain circumstances it will act in the same way in relevantly similar circumstances, the range would also include other propositions which are simply part of a stable background of information which we bring to our enquiries, but which we can imagine coming to reject without overturning the very possibility of gaining an understanding of nature. Examples of the latter might be the proposition that scientific textbooks can be trusted and, in Wittgenstein's time, the proposition that everyone has always been on or near the surface of the earth.

Even those of us who have no commitment to foundationalism are apt to feel nervous about allowing entrenched assumptions to have a normative role. After all, we are inclined to say, entrenched assumptions can just be prejudices or dogmas. Considerations of this sort help to account for a kind of tacit foundationalism which sometimes influences those who do not subscribe to any articulated foundationalist theory and which manifests itself in judgements to the effect that beliefs are irrational or otherwise open to censure unless the believer has adequate grounds in support of the proposition believed.

One might be tempted to try out transcendental arguments on behalf of some at least of those propositions which Wittgenstein would regard as being normative. The aim of deploying such arguments might be to show that the propositions in question are presuppositions of modes of thinking to which we are unavoidably committed, such as forming generalizations about the behaviour of substances on the basis of tests of samples of these substances under various conditions. The hope then would be that we could by these means justify our accepting, for instance, the proposition about the uniform behaviour of substances mentioned above, while leaving out in the cold prejudices and dogmas that happen to be deeply entrenched in the inherited background. Whatever might be said about particular transcendental arguments there is little reason to suppose that this sort of strategy will succeed. In the first place, while arguments of this type may bring to light important propositions on which we tacitly rely, it is not clear how they are supposed to justify our accepting them. What they show, if anything, is that so long as we think in such-and-such a way we must take such-and-such propositions to be true. Even if we cannot imagine not thinking in the way specified it is difficult to see how this shows that we may with propriety accept the propositions to which the way of thinking commits us. Secondly, the strategy presupposes that if the propositions cannot be established by argument then their acceptance cannot be justified and would on that account be open to censure. This might after all be so, but merely to assume it to be so begs the question against the epistemological perspective towards which Wittgenstein seemed to be working.

Two related considerations seem to me to speak powerfully in favour of a view such as Wittgenstein's. First, it seems accurately to reflect our ordinary evaluative practice, at any rate, when we are not doing philosophy or attacking ideologies we do not like. It is easy to challenge those who have views we do not accept to give us some reason for thinking them true, and then, when they cannot or the reasons given seem feeble, to jump in triumphantly with the charge that to hold such views is in some way illegitimate. Sometimes this manœuvre is justified, but it is clear nevertheless that in all our reasoning and thinking we presuppose with others a vast range of propositions for which we neither have nor think we need grounds. This includes many propositions for which grounds could in principle be obtained as well as others, like the evidential propositions linking pain behaviour with pain, or Wittgenstein's proposition about the uniform behaviour of substances, where the possibility of obtaining grounds is at the very least problematic. We do seem to use propositions of these various kinds in ways which make it plausible to think that they have for us a normative status in the sense explained.

The other related consideration is that Wittgenstein's view seems to be psychologically realistic in a way that, for instance, foundationalism certainly is not.[8] We cannot account adequately for the ways in which we actually form, maintain, and evaluate beliefs unless we take account of the many groundless beliefs on which we rely. True, it is a further question whether groundless believing is legitimate, but on this it seems we have just two options. We can be sceptics, agreeing that in practice we do rely on groundless beliefs, but drawing the consequence that beliefs which depend on groundless beliefs are not justified. Or we can tailor our account of the conditions of justification to reflect our actual evaluative practice, in which case, it seems to me, we have to acknowledge the legitimacy of having and relying on groundless beliefs. The approach to justification which I have been sketching is in line with the second option. The issue of scepticism will be taken up in the next chapter.

In the sections which follow I shall develop further the position we have arrived at and defuse some objections to it.

6.3. *Legitimate Belief, Competence, and Rationality*

To possess a concept is to be competent with respect to the inference and quasi-inference patterns by which the concept is individuated. This requires sensitivity to the inferential or quasi-inferential links which instantiate the relevant pattern. (See in particular 2.1.) In this section I shall explore the idea that inference and quasi-inference patterns are associated with requirements which competence alone does not demand that we satisfy. This will turn out to have a bearing on familiar worries over the notion that groundless beliefs may be legitimately held.

Let us say that *P* and *Q* *conflict* if either *P* is an unconditional reason for not-*Q* or *Q* is an unconditional reason for not-*P*. The notion of conflict here is essentially an extension of the notion of inconsistency designed to accommodate the kind of non-deductive inferential links which have loomed large in this book. Now, there is clearly something wrong about accepting

[8] Theories of justification which make inference to a best explanation central are also vulnerable to the charge that they are not psychologically realistic. For such approaches, see Harman (1973) and Lycan (1988). For some relevant considerations, see 3.5 above.

propositions which conflict with one another in this sense. Yet we may do so without failing to satisfy any condition of competence with respect to the relevant inference patterns. Competence with respect to an inference pattern *K* requires an ability to recognize inferences which instantiate *K* as legitimate when they come to one's attention. Sensitivity to inferential links instantiating *K* is a matter of being prepared to take such links into account so far as the recognitional capacity just described enables one to do so. Now having such a capacity does not guarantee that where there is a series of legitimate inferential steps from *P* to not-*Q* one will be aware of this and so not accept both *P* and *Q*. You may easily be unaware that *Q* conflicts with *P* although were you confronted with the steps from *P* to not-*Q* you would appreciate that they were legitimate. The conclusion to be drawn here, I suggest, is that inferential competence does not require ideal rationality. It is a requirement of ideal rationality that you do not accept propositions which conflict with one another. Yet accepting conflicting propositions may be no failure of competence. This is important in reflecting on normative propositions. There is nothing in the notion of a normative proposition which excludes the possibility that there are conflicts between the normative propositions of a perspective. Indeed, if the notion did exclude that possibility it would be useless in the analysis of belief systems. The notion is meant to apply to the contents of background beliefs which are treated as beyond dispute, but there is nothing to say that such beliefs are always internally coherent. Bearing in mind that mastery of a perspective involves the acceptance of its constituent normative propositions this has an important consequence. It may be that mastery of a perspective requires you to accept propositions *P* and *Q*, while ideal rationality requires you to withhold acceptance from at least one of them.

These considerations demand further reflection on the conditions under which propositions may legitimately be taken for granted. Sometimes it is legitimate to take a proposition for granted because we are justified in thinking it true. I have been arguing that it can also be legitimate to take for granted propositions which are normative in the sense explained. But what if accepting some normative proposition involves failing to satisfy an ideal rationality requirement like the requirement not to accept conflicting propositions? Clearly this could happen if normative propositions may conflict with one another.

The strongest response to this problem would be to say that accepting a proposition is not legitimate if it contributes to your failing to satisfy some ideal rationality requirement. But this would be far too restrictive. Think first of the case in which your believing *P* is legitimate because justified. In that case it may well be that you also accept some other proposition conflicting with *P*. Accepting both these propositions leads to your failing to satisfy a requirement of ideal rationality, yet for all that you may be justified in believing *P*. Suppose now that two propositions which are normative for you conflict. The mere fact that they are in conflict does not show that at least one of them is accepted illegitimately. The legitimacy of our beliefs is a function of our perspective and that may well not be fully coherent. However, if it comes to our notice that two propositions which are normative for us are in conflict then it would clearly be illegitimate to accept both. So unless adequate grounds emerge for retaining belief in one rather than the other one should suspend belief in either. The thought here is that known breaches of ideal rationality requirements may not be tolerated and it suggests a general constraint on the legitimacy of belief: A belief is not legitimate if having it contributes to a breach in an ideal rationality requirement of which the subject is aware and abandoning it is required in order to avoid that breach.

I have been speaking of conflicts among normative propositions but obviously there may be conflicts between normative propositions and other non-normative propositions which we accept. The role of a legitimately accepted normative proposition dictates that we reject propositions which conflict with it. But we could come to have adequate grounds for accepting a proposition which conflicts with a normative proposition. Thus, if all the facts speak for people having been to the moon it would be crazy to hold on to the proposition that no one has ever been to the moon even if it has had a normative role for us. Note, however, that the requirement to avoid conflict does not of itself dictate that we should abandon the normative proposition rather than the proposition which conflicts with it. There seems to be another ideal rationality requirement in play and it is something like this: Do not believe a proposition if there are adequate grounds for thinking it false. There can be adequate grounds for believing a proposition which conflicts with a normative proposition and thus adequate grounds for rejecting the normative proposition. It might seem that this latter claim could be resisted. Why not take the line that if a proposition conflicts with a normative proposition then there cannot be adequate grounds for thinking it true? Well, if we do want to include among possible normative propositions the proposition that no one has ever been to the moon this line is going to be heroic indeed. If it is to be sustainable it needs to be made plausible by a systematic account of reasons which will explain why the weight given to the normative proposition must always override that given to the considerations which support the proposition which conflicts with it. No such account is in prospect.

The two requirements discussed thus far are by no means the only requirements of ideal rationality. Suppose you are firmly convinced of the truth of some highly speculative hypothesis for which there is no evidence whatsoever, so far as you or anyone else knows. Returning again to the deer track example of 2.4, the proposition might be that alien beings from another planet occasionally come to earth and create tracks identical in form to those produced by a familiar species of deer. Let us call this hypothesis *H*. Intuitively, we should regard your believing *H* as some kind of intellectual failing, but as yet we have no explanation of why this is so. I assume that *H* is neither a normative proposition nor one which you would be justified in believing. But we lack an explanation of why this should matter. Our conditions of justification show that you would not be justified in believing *H*, but they do not explain what is wrong with having an unjustified belief. Indeed, my interpretation of the Basis condition allows for legitimate beliefs which are not justified, in the sense of deriving justification from beliefs or experiences. Moreover, accepting *H* need not result in a breach of either of the rationality requirements considered so far. What seems to be missing is a grounding requirement, that is, a requirement to the effect that one should not believe to be true a proposition like *H* unless one believes it on adequate grounds, where that means that one has adequate grounds for believing it and does so because one has adequate grounds. The grounding requirement is in effect the requirement to believe a proposition like *H* only if one is derivatively justified in doing so, for to believe on adequate grounds is, surely, just to be derivatively justified. Believing *H* would be in breach of this requirement.

It seems that we do recognize some kind of grounding requirement but now we have what threatens to be a problem for the epistemological framework which I have been developing. The framework allows that there can be beliefs whose contents are normative propositions and which are groundless. How can it be legitimate to take normative propositions for granted if we are subject to a grounding requirement? The way out of our problem is to appreciate that although we are subject to a grounding requirement it is of limited scope. Let us consider the speculative proposition *H* again. We would be puzzled by your believing *H*, since we do not believe it and you have given us no reason to think that we should. Our puzzle here is related to the thought that belief aims at truth.[9] Not only are beliefs evaluable with respect to truth and falsity, it is intrinsic to believing that we aim to believe only what is true. That aim generates the rationality requirements to avoid believing conflicting propositions and avoid believing a proposition if there are adequate grounds for thinking it false. It also generates a grounding requirement. We have an interest in ensuring that when propositions we do not already believe come up for our consideration we do not believe them true unless we have adequate grounds for thinking them true. To believe whatever takes our fancy would not be consistent with aiming to believe only what is true. That is why *H* is unacceptable. But to account for what is awry about accepting *H* we do not need to postulate an unqualified grounding requirement. Accepting *H* would be ruled out by a qualified grounding requirement along the following lines: If a proposition *P* which you do not already believe comes up for your consideration do not believe it unless you have adequate grounds for doing so.

The worry which led to these last considerations was that accepting normative propositions groundlessly might fall foul of some grounding requirement. Clearly such acceptance is not

[9] See Bernard Williams (1970) and (1978), ch. 2. Compare Alston (1985).

proscribed by our qualified grounding requirement since it only applies to propositions we do not already believe.

The qualified grounding requirement and the requirement not to believe a proposition if there are adequate grounds for thinking it false should go some way towards allaying fears that the view of normative propositions for which I am arguing licenses either credulity or dogmatism. The former requirement rules out credulity while the latter rules out dogmatism conceived as holding on to beliefs in the face of reasons for abandoning them. Yet neither of these requirements nor the requirement to avoid conflict rules out the possibility of legitimately held groundless beliefs.

There is a further problem which may be posed along the following lines. Let it be granted that aiming to believe only what is true generates rationality requirements. How can it be that this aim generates less than an unqualified grounding requirement? We need to address this matter but I shall defer its discussion until the final chapter where it will be considered in the context of a general treatment of scepticism.

6.4. *More on Perspectives*

In developing an account of perspectives which echoes the themes from Wittgenstein noticed earlier one might be tempted, and encouraged by some of Wittgenstein's own remarks, to think of differences in perspective on the model of differences in the outlooks of geographically distinct and culturally diverse societies. I think it is fairly clear that this way of thinking is misleading. It overlooks the continuity in perspectives across geographically distinct societies, even where these are culturally very different. It also overlooks the differences in perspectives within societies.

Terms like 'society' are notoriously vague. Here, when I speak of society I shall be thinking of, for example, something like British society or United States society or Malaysian society. In other words, I shall think of a society as a population which occupies some geographical region and within which there is a high degree of social interaction and mutual interdependence. Political integration is perhaps not essential, but will be present in many if not most cases. The same may be said for shared language. We don't want the Swiss to end up not having a society. Also, there may be various significant cultural differences within a society. These points granted, it is evident that diversity of perspective within a society is commonplace. Among those which naturally spring to mind are differences linked with religion.

Christians, for example, have a theological perspective which is certainly not shared by everyone in the societies to which they belong. But Christians share with others perspectives which include various logical concepts, a host of descriptive concepts and associated presuppositions, as well as multifarious propositions about food and drink, clothes, housing, transport, government, money, etiquette, sex, weather, communication, history, geography, health, medicine, and the like. Now, if we are interested in understanding the attitudes and modes of thought of Christians it is clear that we have to take into account not just those of their beliefs which have a theological content, for how these beliefs function in relation to thought and action will depend to a large extent on the non-theological beliefs which Christians have. If you think that a person at some point in history was inspired by God you must also have many beliefs about that person which others who do not have your theological beliefs might share, but without which you could not have your distinctively theological beliefs about the person in question. This being so it is better not to think of a Christian perspective as what is left over when you subtract the mundane from the overall perspective of a Christian. Rather, any Christian perspective will include a mundane perspective though, of course, there are mundane perspectives without the overlay of a Christian or any other religious perspective.

It might be felt that this way of looking at things is wrong in assuming that mundane perspectives may be incorporated within, yet detachable from, religious ones. The worry would be that this ignores the extent to which religious 'overlays' permeate thinking about mundane things. But the detachability claim is actually a very modest one. It would take a great deal of heavy and, I think, dubious theory to dislodge it. I do not deny that religious perspectives involve beliefs about the religious significance of mundane things. Catholics, for instance, appear to believe that in certain contexts bread and wine can, in some sense, be the body and blood of Christ, and Christians in general may sometimes think that people have been saved from injury or death by the hand of God. Even so, Catholics share with others commonplace beliefs about bread and wine outside of ritual contexts, and Christians in general share with others commonplace beliefs about dangers to life and limb. It is simply false that distinctively religious concepts enter into the contents of every belief that the religious believer has.

For the detachability claim to be true all that is required is that for every Christian perspective *v* there is a perspective which *v* incorporates and which could be shared by others who do not share *v*. It does not require that there is some perspective such that all perspectives must incorporate it. Nor does it require that every perspective must incorporate a perspective whose constituent concepts are all observational in some strict sense and whose constituent propositions have only observational concepts as descriptive ingredients.

Evaluations of people's beliefs with respect to legitimacy must be made by reference to their own perspective, and thus to the concept-exhibiting inference and quasi-inference patterns and the normative propositions by which they are governed. This is a consequence of the regulative approach to epistemology which I have adopted. Obviously perspectives may vary in respect of their constituent concepts as well as in respect of their constituent normative propositions. A couple of examples will serve to illustrate how variations in normative propositions bear on the evaluation of beliefs with respect to justification, and thus also with respect to legitimacy.

Aristarchus of Samos, in the third century BC, apparently held that the earth rotates about its axis and revolves around the sun (*T*).[10] Little is known about why he took this view. There are relatively few references to it in ancient literature and it seems not to have been taken seriously by other astronomers. It is arguable that, against the background of the perspectives available at the time, there were adequate grounds for rejecting *T*. Assuming that the earth revolves around the sun then, given the vast distances which it would traverse and the sort of

[10] See Toulmin and Goodfield (1963) and the literature referred to there.

distances it was plausible to suppose the stars could be from the earth, while still being visible, it was to be expected that there would be a visible parallax of the stars, that is, a visible displacement in their relative positions as the earth moves across space. No parallax was detectable. Also, if the earth rotated about its axis then, given a certain natural assumption, it should be expected that things near to but not in contact with the surface of the earth, like clouds or projectiles, would never appear to move eastwards, the direction of rotation. The natural assumption was that such things would be, as it were, left behind as the earth rapidly rotates towards the east. But evidently such things can be observed to move eastwards. So there was reason to reject Aristarchus' theory in that it conflicted with observable facts. The theory is not, of course, logically incompatible with the fact that there is no visible stellar parallax and that things near to but not in contact with the surface of the earth can be detected to move eastwards. It conflicts with the facts only given certain auxiliary assumptions which we now believe to be false. Using instruments stellar parallax can now be detected and we have no difficulty in conceiving of the stars being so far away that parallax is not detectable by unaided sight. Nor do we expect things which are not in contact with the earth to be moving westwards as the earth rotates eastwards, for we have a dynamical theory which accounts for how they can move eastwards. But it could be that in Aristarchus' time it was normative for astronomers that the stars could not be anything like as far away as is required by Aristarchus' theory and normative that if the earth were in motion in the way required for diurnal rotation then a point on its surface would 'leave behind' any objects above and not in contact with it. In fact, it seems quite likely that the theory was not taken seriously just because these propositions were normative for most of those who considered these matters.

The other example is from Durkheim. Drawing on ethnographic data provided by Spencer and Gillen, Durkheim describes some features of the thought and practice of native Australians in the Witchetty Grub clan.[11] Members of this clan, a branch of the Arunta tribe, apparently thought that the

[11] Durkheim (1976), pp. 326 ff.

scattering of dust which had come from certain sacred rocks would ensure the reproductive success of the local witchetty grub. So each year they would accept a proposition like *G*, 'This year there will be plenty of grubs because dust from these rocks has been appropriately scattered.' For us the connection between the scattering of dust and the reproduction of some species is obscure to say the least. But the connection becomes intelligible once we take into account that the rocks in question were believed to have a special association with ancient ancestors of the clan and that the grubs were conceived as being in a relation of kinship with the clan. According to Witchetty Grub mythology the ancestors endowed the rocks with special powers which were carried by the dust and were responsible for the fertilization of the grub. The story, in effect, had a normative role for the clan.

We think there are good grounds for accepting *T* and rejecting *G*. Nevertheless, I take it that we are prepared to allow that not-*T* and *G* could each have been legitimately inferred from the relevant background assumptions together with appropriate empirical data. So believing not-*T* or *G* to be true would be intelligible in a context in which the relevant background assumptions were held and the relevant empirical data thought to obtain. But, more importantly, believing not-*T* and believing *G* in the contexts in question could have been justified and for that reason legitimate. If the background assumptions had a normative role and could legitimately be taken for granted there would have been in these contexts adequate grounds for believing not-*T* and *G* respectively. Whether any such beliefs actually were justified depends on historical facts which we need not go into. The important thing is that in contexts such as seem to have obtained they very well might have been.[12]

Such a view obviously places a great deal of weight on the

[12] William Newton-Smith (1982) notes that beliefs which we find bizarre can often be rendered more intelligible in the light of relevant background beliefs. He rightly stresses that even where there are differences in background beliefs there must be similarities in modes of reasoning and that unless we can discern modes of reasoning in a group which are like our own we cannot even make sense of their having beliefs. However, I differ from Newton-Smith in thinking that the contents of background beliefs have a normative role whereby they partially determine what counts as a reasonable or justified belief on the part of those who share these beliefs.

notion of a normative proposition. I have already argued that it would be a mistake to suppose that the view sanctions dogmatism if by that is meant clinging on to a belief in the face of good reasons to abandon it. So far as we know the contemporaries of Aristarchus had no good reason to abandon their belief in the background propositions which got in the way of their taking his hypothesis seriously. Presumably at the time they were investigated by Spencer and Gillen the Witchetty Grub people had no reason to abandon their background beliefs about the propagation of the witchetty grub. It is quite possible that in both cases holding to the crucial background propositions was not proscribed by any requirement of rationality.

Having said that it is worth considering whether there are not other requirements of rationality which would place further constraints on the rational acceptance of normative propositions. Here is a line of thought which suggests that there are.

Suppose we think of the fundamental concepts and propositions of Christianity or, more precisely, some version of traditional Christianity, as forming part of a perspective in the way already outlined. This is plausible since ordinary Christians by and large do not believe what they do about God, the world, and humankind because they think that there are adequate grounds for belief. Rather, they come to be governed by a Christian perspective as a result of being brought up among, or falling in with, others who believe. It may be part of the perspective that there is evidence of the existence of God provided by the beauty and intricate structures of nature, by what is conceived to be the history of God's dealings with humankind, and by the sense which many Christians have of being guided or sustained or judged by God. But believing that there is evidence does not imply believing because one believes there is evidence. As often as not the basic doctrinal stance is accepted before people encounter ideas about evidence of the wisdom and glory of God. Even when these ideas are encountered they do not always have a sustaining role in relation to the basic doctrinal stance. Undergraduate lectures on the problems besetting traditional arguments for the existence of God sometimes convince Christians that the arguments are unsound, but only rarely do Christians draw the conclusion that they should abandon their faith.

Now with regard to many issues on which Christianity takes a stand there are alternative views, that is, views on the issues conflicting with the Christian view. For example, traditional Christianity has a view on the factors which explain the course of ancient Israelite history and the rise and development of the Christian Church. The view is, roughly speaking, that things happened in the way they did because the hand of God was at work nudging the course of events in one direction rather than another. Any such view conflicts with historical accounts which purport to offer adequate explanations of the events in question, so far as they are known, in purely secular terms. For Christian accounts along the lines just indicated have it that events would not have taken the course they did but for the hand of God, while the secular accounts deny that this is so. Somewhat similar conflicts occur between Christians and evolutionary theorists on the matter of how human beings come to be the way they are.

Those who are attracted by the alternatives to the Christian view on the issues mentioned need not think that Christianity is refuted, for they need not hold that there are adequate grounds for accepting the alternative view. They may confine themselves to the claim that the Christian view is not mandatory since these alternatives are at least as plausible. Let us suppose for the sake of argument that accepting the Christian view on the issues in the face of the availability of alternatives need not breach the requirement not to believe a proposition if there are adequate grounds for thinking it false. It is arguable none the less that *groundless* acceptance of the Christian view would be in some sense irrational. The thought here is that the very existence of plausible alternatives makes it irrational to continue to accept the Christian view unless it can be shown to be better than the alternatives. The relevant rationality requirement would be something like this: If a proposition *P* presents a view on some issue and there are plausible alternatives to *P* on that issue then do not accept *P* unless you have reason to prefer it to the alternatives.

It might be thought that this requirement has little bite since Christians could simply deny the plausibility of the alternatives. Judgements of plausibility may legitimately be influenced by background beliefs. So why should the Christian not simply judge, say, purely secular accounts of history, to be implausible on the ground that they conflict with the fundamental tenets of Christianity? Well, certainly taking this line would not necessarily conflict with the requirement not to believe a proposition if there are adequate grounds for thinking it false, and there may be contexts in which it is legitimate. But, I contend, it would be illegitimate in a context in which the alternative view is made plausible by other things the Christian believes. Plausibility is plausibility relative to certain considerations. Even if the alternative view is not plausible relative to fundamental Christian assumptions it may be plausible relative to other assumptions which the Christian shares with those who favour the alternative view. If the issue in question is the history of the early Church the assumptions may have to do with the explanation of human behaviour and the sorts of factors which operate to account for the rise of religious movements. If the Christian relies on these assumptions when dealing with ordinary history as opposed to the history which Christians regard as sacred, and if these assumptions make plausible a secular account of the allegedly sacred history, then there is an incoherence in the overall system of beliefs which the Christian holds. This is not to say that the only way to resolve the incoherence would be to abandon the Christian view. The point is rather that to hold on to the Christian account of the stretch of history in question without grounds for preferring it to the secular alternative would be irrational.

I am inclined to think that rationality does impose upon us something like the requirement to eliminate alternatives. Neither this nor the other ideal rationality requirements considered make groundless beliefs as such irrational. But these requirements do help to account for how it can be reasonable to abandon belief in a proposition which has had a normative role. This is important for it reinforces a point made at the end of the last section. To countenance legitimately groundless beliefs is not to license dogmatism or credulity.[13]

[13] Wright in his (1980), pp. 415 and 419 ff., notes the problem of distinguishing statements having normative status from dogma. He is specifically concerned with statements to which we attach necessity, but the problem is a general one.

7

Scepticism

7.1. *The Suspension of Belief*

The topic of scepticism has been undergoing something of a revival of late.[1] It is not difficult to understand its continuing fascination. There is a clash between our lack of concern with scepticism for all practical and, outside of philosophy, even theoretical purposes, and the difficulty of satisfying ourselves that the sceptic's challenges can be adequately met. In this final chapter I shall briefly explore some of the issues drawing on materials supplied earlier in the book. I shall confine my attention to beliefs concerning the world at large, including our own immediate environment and the people within it.

Right at the start we are faced with the problem of stating what scepticism is. One possibility is that scepticism is not so much a thesis as an attitude of mind in which belief is suspended on all matters. Apparently, global suspension of belief was regarded by ancient sceptics as the way to a tranquil life.[2] It is no small problem to conceive of what it would be to adopt such a stance.

The nub of the problem is the link between intentional action and belief. We cannot act intentionally in familiar ways unless we have beliefs about the world around us. You can intentionally go to buy food in some location only if you have beliefs to the effect that food can be bought at that location, that you can get there by such-and-such a route using such-and-such means, and so forth. Suspending all belief about the environment would therefore require one to abstain from intentional actions

[1] See e.g. Burnyeat (1983), Penelhum (1983), Stroud (1984), Wright (1985), Nagel (1986).

[2] See e.g. Burnyeat (1980) and Penelhum (1983). I was provoked into a reaction to this sort of scepticism by a paper given by Jonathan Barnes in the Stirling Philosophy Department in spring 1987.

which depend on beliefs about the environment, and then the problem is to see not just why anyone should wish to live such a life, but, more significantly, how with such abstinence one could make one's way through the world and interact in normal human ways with other people.

To meet this problem it might be suggested that a genuine sceptic would never act intentionally, but would be carried along by custom and habit.[3] Certainly, we do engage in habitual routines. Think of walking a route to or from work each day. You may go along on automatic pilot, as it were, absorbed in thoughts that have nothing to do with the scenes you encounter. But even here your action is thoroughly intentional. You aim to get to work or to go home. You have beliefs about the locations of the university and your home, about why you are going to either place, and about how to reach these places from where you start out. Your routine walk is not immune to changes of belief concerning these matters. If you suddenly remember that the university library is closed for the day and you were going in with the sole purpose of checking references there you might well turn back. Sometimes we do things unintentionally. Suppose that your department changes its location. Shortly after the change you may find yourself from time to time going to the old location out of habit. Here you certainly do not intend to go to the old location. But there are intentions in the background, for instance, to go to the department. A life in which every action was like your habitually and unintentionally going to the old location, if coherently conceivable at all, would not be recognizably human. It is hardly a life which anyone could seriously wish to lead, yet it seems to be all that is available to a being who lacked beliefs.

To reinforce the point suppose that you are thirsty and you have a visual experience of a glass of water. You reach out to pick up the glass. Can we make sense of your doing this deliberately, and thus in some sense intentionally, without your

[3] The rule of life recommended by Sextus Empiricus speaks of being guided by Nature, the constraint of the passions, the tradition of law and customs, and instruction in the arts. See Sextus Empiricus (1933), i. 23–4, and the discussions already referred to by Burnyeat and Penelhum. The suggestion seems to be that we allow ourselves to be carried along by those dispositions we have in virtue of our native constitution and acquired habits. However, as I point out below, it is implausible to suppose that living in this way could be intention-free.

believing that a glass of water is in front of you? I think not. You want to bring it about that you are drinking a glass of water. Anything you do intentionally to satisfy this desire must be conceived by you as being relevant, and thus at least likely to be instrumental, to its satisfaction. If you do not believe that a glass is actually there then you could hardly conceive of your reaching out for a glass in this way. What if you just believe that there is some chance that a glass of water is there? In that case we have some inclination, I think, to regard you not as intending to pick up the glass but merely as hoping to pick up the glass. Furthermore, believing there is some chance that a glass of water is there is still believing something about the world, and that would be ruled out by a total suspension of belief.

Even if it could be made plausible that a being with no beliefs could negotiate the world there would remain the problem of understanding how we could make the transition from having beliefs to having none. Whatever might be said about the intelligibility of abandoning all beliefs there is no realistic prospect of ever doing so. A different approach is called for. We need to consider why the possibility of a global suspension of belief should have been taken seriously at all. The motivation is supplied by doubts as to whether any of our beliefs about the world around us are legitimate. On the face of it there is an intelligible position in which such beliefs continue to be held, but in which belief is suspended as to whether any are legitimate. I shall call this global scepticism with regard to the legitimacy of beliefs. As stated it is a stance rather than a thesis. It is a stance which the global sceptic invites us to adopt in the light of sceptical considerations about the legitimacy of our beliefs. I shall focus on scepticism about whether any of our beliefs are truly justified and thus on that account legitimate. Given the views developed in previous chapters it is clear that problems having to do with groundless beliefs will not be far behind.

At this point, though, we need to reflect on how sceptical considerations about justification are supposed to relate to the suspension of belief with regard to whether any of our beliefs are justified. The sceptical considerations might be taken to establish a sceptical thesis, namely that none of our beliefs about the world about us is justified. If sceptics think there are good grounds for adopting the sceptical thesis then this obviously would place limits on just how sceptical they can be about our modes of reasoning. They must think that we can reason well enough to be able to appreciate the strength of the sceptical thesis even though our beliefs about the world about us are not justified. There arises then the question whether this position is coherent; in particular, whether the sceptical thesis leaves room for the possibility that we could be justified in accepting it. Essentially the same problem arises if sceptical considerations about reasoning and justification are conceived merely as grounds for doubt about whether any of our beliefs about the world around us are justified, rather than grounds for believing that no such beliefs are justified. It is not a trivial matter to decide whether sceptics can cope with these problems. So long as scepticism is restricted to beliefs about the world, the obvious response would be to argue that we can know a priori that the required considerations about justification are true even if we suspend belief on whether any of our beliefs about the world are justified. If there are real difficulties here sceptics have the option of falling back on the idea that the sceptical considerations do not so much justify as causally induce an attitude of doubt with regard to the justification of our beliefs. But then if the sceptical considerations do not have this effect on the rest of us the sceptic could hardly complain that they ought to.

We can set out to refute global scepticism with regard to justification only if it contains some positive claim about justification. The claim might be that none of our beliefs about the world are justified or that there are considerations which cast doubt on whether any of our beliefs about the world is justified. Or it might just be that our thinking about justification is incoherent and so we ought to suspend our evaluative practice. Any such claim would be recognizably sceptical and would give us something to bite into.

7.2. *Crude Sceptical Strategies*

We operate with what might be called a *system of justification*. A system of justification comprises a set of conditions of justified belief, such as set out in Chapters 2 and 4, interpreted in the light of a perspective, as conceived in Chapter 6. The conditions of justified belief are not tied to any specific perspective. They tell us, for example, that a belief that *p* derives its justification from beliefs that *q*, *r*, . . . only if *q*, *r*, . . . constitute an unconditional reason for *p*. But to know what counts as an unconditional reason we need to know the perspective of the subject. The relevant perspective interprets the conditions of justified belief and thus gives us the system of justification relevant to the appraisal of the subject's beliefs.

For the purposes of exploring philosophical scepticism we may think of ourselves as sharing a system of justification. This over-simplifies the actual situation in view of the diversity of perspectives, but that is of no consequence. There is enough overlap in our perspectives to make the differences irrelevant, when what is at stake is not any particular person's beliefs, but a whole outlook on the world which we share. With these caveats in mind let us call our shared system of justification, the *S*-system. Beliefs which that system counts as being justified are *S*-justified.

I want to focus initially on a sceptical strategy which takes the following general form. Certain conditions on justified belief are set out and it is argued that since none of the beliefs which are *S*-justified satisfies the conditions none of these beliefs is truly justified. The effect of the strategy is to suggest that the *S*-system is not properly regarded as a system of justification at all. To mount this strategy the sceptic must have some conception of what the 'right' conditions of justification are.

There are various possible conceptions of the 'right conditions'. One conception requires that justifying reasons, that is reasons in virtue of which our Rational Connection conditions (2.1, 4.3) could be satisfied, must be conclusive. The condition *JUS2*' (2.1) requires that justifying propositional reasons should be unconditional and not that they should be conclusive. To recap: *q*, *r*, . . . constitute an unconditional reason for *p* if and only if *p* is inferable from *q*, *r*, . . . without further ado; *q*, *r*, . . . constitute a conclusive reason for *p* if and only if it is not possible that *q*, *r*, . . . are true while *p* is false. A theme of previous chapters has been that there are important types of reason which are unconditional yet inconclusive. One type comprises the reasons which bear on the ascription of pain to someone on the basis of pain behaviour (3.2). The sceptic who takes the view that justifying propositional reasons must be conclusive will not regard as truly justified ascriptions of pain to others which hinge on inconclusive reasons. Such sceptics will also look askance at the conditions under which *E*-beliefs are *S*-justified. According to the theory of Chapter 4 the justification of *E*-beliefs turns on a special class of reasons which I called experiential reasons. In a sense closely parallel to that pertaining to propositional reasons these reasons are both unconditional yet inconclusive, and so, according to the sceptic we are now considering, not fit to count as justifying reasons. If this is right then given the fundamental role of these beliefs it is plausible that scepticism about justification extends to all beliefs about the world held on grounds.

Another condition on justified belief which the sceptic might deploy is that a belief that *p* cannot be justificationally dependent on any belief which is not itself justified. (Recall that to be justified is to be derivatively justified.) I rejected any such condition precisely in order to allow that beliefs could be justificationally dependent on groundless beliefs. Normative propositions may be legitimately taken for granted and thus groundless beliefs to the effect that some normative proposition is true may satisfy the Basis condition *JUS4*. But if that is not so and all basis beliefs have to be justified then very many beliefs would never be justified.

The 'right conditions' I have mentioned do not exhaust those which a sceptic might deploy. They are particularly germane if inconclusive reasons and groundless beliefs are as fundamental to the *S*-system as I have suggested, but there are conceivable sceptical strategies which turn on other conditions. What is important for our purposes is the very idea that sceptical conclusions can be derived using conditions of justified belief which are at odds with the system of justification with which we actually operate.

A familiar way of developing a sceptical argument relies on the indisputable point that where the grounds we have for accepting a proposition are inconclusive they do not rule out all the alternatives to the proposition. I may believe there is a cup before me in response to a current experience of a cup. The conditions for the belief to be justified, as spelled out by the *S*-

system, may be satisfied, yet their being satisfied is consistent with the possibility that there is no cup before me and that my experience is explained by manipulation of my brain-patterns of which I am completely unaware. The situation is one in which there are countervailing facts with respect to there being a cup before me, but for all that I might, within the standards of the *S*-system, legitimately take for granted that there are none. The sceptic, however, suggests that if you were truly justified in believing that a cup is there you would have to have established specifically that your experience is not caused by manipulation of your brain-patterns. In ordinary situations you would make no attempt to do any such thing and it is at least doubtful that you could do so even if you tried.

As it stands this type of argument is question-begging. What does seem to be a necessary condition of your being justified in believing that a cup is there in the circumstances described is that you may legitimately overlook the possibility that your experience results from manipulation of your brain-patterns. The *S*-system permits you to overlook this possibility since, in the ordinary course of events, it is not a live alternative to there being a cup before you. (Recall here the discussion in 2.4.) In order to derive the conclusion that your belief is not justified the sceptic needs to assume that overlooking outlandish alternatives to a proposition is incompatible with being justified in believing it true. To deploy such an assumption is just to adopt a strong condition on justified belief which is at odds with the *S*-system.

A closely related way of generating scepticism about justification is via the following plausible principle: If you are justified in believing that p and justified in believing that p entails q, then you would be justified in believing that q.[4] This principle was not operative in the discussion of the last example, since there being a cup before you does not entail that your brain is not being manipulated so that you have an experience of a cup before you. But here is a version of a classic case to which the principle is relevant. My being in Bridge of Allan entails that it is not the case that I am a brain in a vat on Alpha Centauri. The suggestion is that I am not justified in believing that I am not a

[4] In recent years closure principles analogous to this have received attention as a result of Nozick (1981). Nozick's discussion is of a closure principle for knowledge.

brain in a vat in Alpha Centauri, since all my experiences could be just as they are even if I were in that unfortunate situation. So by the closure principle I am not justified in believing that I am in Bridge of Allan. I am inclined to accept the closure principle. But assuming it is correct the sceptic's conclusion is only delivered on the assumption that I am not justified in believing that I am not a brain in a vat on Alpha Centauri. The sceptic adopts this assumption on the grounds that all my experiences could be just as they are if I were a brain in a vat on Alpha Centauri. The grounds are, in other words, that my experiences do not logically exclude my being a brain in a vat on Alpha Centauri. But why are these grounds relevant? They would only be relevant if I could not be justified in believing that *p* unless my experiences logically exclude the possibility that not-*p*, and that condition is plainly at odds with the *S*-system. So this strategy too depends on strong assumptions about the right conditions of justification. In this particular case the sceptic overlooks the possibility that I could be justified in believing that I am not a brain in a vat on Alpha Centauri since I am justified in believing I am in Bridge of Allan and justified in believing that my being in Bridge of Allan entails that I am not a brain in a vat on Alpha Centauri.[5] A way of trying to block such a possibility is to assume that I would not be justified in believing that I am in Bridge of Allan unless I had *checked out* that I am not a brain in a vat on Alpha Centauri, independently of what leads me to believe that I am in Bridge of Allan. But it is far from clear that our ordinary ways of thinking about justification, as captured by the *S*-system, impose any such requirement. So again the line of argument proposed looks like a version of the strategy presently under consideration. A strong condition on justified belief, which is out of tune with the *S*-system, is being used to criticize the *S*-system.

Somewhat unfairly, I shall call sceptical strategies of the sort described, *crude strategies*. There is a response to such strategies which turns on a conception of what determines that a particular account of the conditions of justified belief is correct or incorrect. According to this conception an account is correct if

[5] I have the impression that Michael Williams made a somewhat similar point in connection with the corresponding principle for knowledge in a talk given in the Stirling Philosophy Department in spring 1987 and in another given to the Realism and Reason conference in St. Andrews in spring 1988.

and only if (by and large) beliefs which we would ordinarily and on careful reflection think of as justified satisfy the stated conditions and beliefs which we would ordinarily and on careful reflection think of as unjustified fail to satisfy the stated conditions. Perhaps there can be difficult cases in which we should stick with the proposed account even though our evaluations clash with it. If so the account must make it plausible that the evaluations are awry rather than the proposed account. This sort of conception takes it that the scrutiny of careful evaluations of actual or imagined cases will reveal the conditions under which beliefs are justified. But there is nothing question-begging about that. The aim is to devise an account of the conditions on justified belief and there is nothing else to go on in supplying such an account than our best evaluative practice. This is the procedure which I followed in previous chapters. It is a procedure by which we come to appreciate, for instance, that beliefs can be justified even though the reasons for holding them are inconclusive. We do not thereby discover anything which vindicates our reliance on inconclusive reasons. We simply come to realize that our system of justification allows for reliance on reasons of that type.

The conception just sketched, or something very like it, is widely, though not universally, accepted.[6] If it is along the right lines then a response to crude sceptical strategies is at hand. The conditions on justified belief which the sceptic proposes are at odds with our best evaluative practice. The sceptic must agree with this since his scepticism springs from his view that the standards implicit in our evaluative practice are inadequate. But the problem which now emerges for the sceptic's position is that there is no adequate rationale for the conditions on justified belief which he proposes, and no prospect of providing one given the way in which accounts of the conditions of justified belief have to be supported. So crude sceptical strategies are undermined. They do not so much as cast doubt on whether any of our beliefs are justified since they rely on assumptions about justified belief which have no proper grounding.

[6] Philosophers adopt the proposed approach even when they do not talk about it. For explicit discussions in connection with induction, see Goodman (1965), ch. 3, and, in a similar vein, Hesse (1974), ch. 4. For more general considerations, see Cohen (1981, 1986).

7.3. *A Sophisticated Sceptical Strategy*

We are liable, and I think we ought, to feel unease at the suggestion that scepticism can be laid to rest simply by rebutting crude sceptical strategies in the manner just outlined. The problem with these strategies is that they rely on assumptions about justification which receive no support from our evaluative practice. The more sophisticated strategy which we shall consider now relies on an assumption which is supposed to be implicit in our ordinary thinking about justification rather than imposed arbitrarily by the sceptic. The assumption is that justification should be *truth-indicative*.

To make this more precise I shall make use of the following notions. A mode of justification is a type of justification involving a particular series of inferential or quasi-inferential steps leading to a particular conclusion, and thus also a particular type of basis. A belief may be said to be *M*-justified if its justification is of the mode *M*. Beliefs which have the same content are instances of the same belief type. A mode of justification pertains to a belief type if instances of that type could have justifications of that mode. For each mode of justification there is just one belief type to which it pertains, determined by the proposition which is the conclusion of the relevant series of inferential and quasi-inferential steps. We can now introduce the notion of truth-indicativeness for a mode of justification *M* as follows.

TI *M* is truth-indicative if and only if the belief type *T* to which *M* pertains is such that instances of *T* which were *M*-justified would more often than not be true.

Note that truth-indicativeness should not be conflated with the notion of truth-conduciveness introduced in 2.4 and 4.3. Truth-conduciveness is a property of inference and quasi-inference patterns. Truth-conducive inference patterns are reliable in that inferences, in the psychological sense, instantiating such a pattern and having true premisses would more often than not have true conclusions. Truth-conducive quasi-inference patterns are reliable in that quasi-inferences, in the psychological sense, instantiating such a pattern, from an experience of an appropriate type, and a true proposition to the effect that there are no relevant countervailing facts, would more often than not have true conclusions. Truth-indicativeness is a property of modes of justification which satisfy all the conditions of the *S*-system.

Sophisticated sceptics propose that truth-indicativeness is a condition of *genuine* justification. Thus we have

JUS(*GEN*) *M* is a mode of genuine justification only if *M* is truth-indicative.

The rationale for *JUS*(*GEN*) lies in a conception of the point of evaluating beliefs with respect to justification. The conception is that justified beliefs are beliefs which are commendable from the point of view of aiming to believe what is true and not to believe what is false. This leads to the thought that a belief which is held on such-and-such grounds will be commendable from this point of view only if holding beliefs on grounds of that sort is a reliable method for realizing the aim of believing only what is true.[7] If the *S*-justification for a belief is of a mode which is not truth-indicative this condition will not be met.

Granted *JUS*(*GEN*) it is a further question whether it can be used in support of an interesting scepticism. Sophisticated sceptics, however, can argue with some plausibility that the *S*-system does not guarantee that *JUS*(*GEN*) is satisfied for the modes of justification which it accommodates.

With regard to some modes of justification countenanced by the *S*-system it seems to be possible that justifications in these modes are not genuine. Consider modes of justification for beliefs which make these beliefs justificationally dependent on groundless beliefs which are in fact false. In this connection it is helpful to recall the discussion of ascriptions of pain in Chapter 3 where we considered inferences from behaviour to pain. There I argued that our practice of applying the concept of pain on behavioural grounds depends on assumptions to the effect that the occurrence of a particular sort of behaviour is strong fallible evidence that the subject is in pain. These assumptions are contingent. Thus, for instance, it is contingent that wincing is strong fallible evidence for pain, for there are possible worlds in which wincing is more often than not caused by something

[7] Compare Alston (1985).

other than pain. It seems possible that there should be some strange syndrome which afflicts certain people so as to make them feign pain in various ways, including wincing, and never reveal to others that they have done so. It also seems to be possible that a majority of people should become afflicted with this syndrome and that a majority should have no knowledge that this is so. Those who are aware that they are afflicted may be unaware that anyone else is. The sceptic may argue with some plausibility that for all we know the actual world is just such a world. Now, take the mode of justification for beliefs that a person is in pain which has the form considered in 3.1 and 3.2 (the form analogous to that which figured in the deer track case) and which relies on the supposed strong fallible evidential link between wincing and pain. Call this mode *W*. Sceptics can point out that, even if the evidential link in question does not obtain, beliefs that a subject is in pain could be *W*-justified. Only one of our conditions of justified belief might seem to be strained by this claim and that is the Basis condition. This was the condition which required that if a belief derives its justification in part from the belief that *p* then it must be legitimate to take it for granted that *p*. But by the standards of the *S*-system it may be that it is legitimate to take it for granted that the evidential link between wincing and pain holds even if the link does not in fact obtain. And surely it could also be legitimate to take for granted that there are no countervailing facts with respect to the subject's being in pain, for people who are unaware of the feigning syndrome have no reason to take it into account. If such a world is indeed possible and our world were such a world then being *W*-justified in believing that a person is in pain would not be a reliable indicator of its being true that the person is in pain. In that case *W*-justification would not be genuine justification.

The sophisticated sceptic might then argue that considerations analogous to those set out for *W*-justification would go through for any mode of justification which involves justificational dependence on groundless beliefs in contingent evidential links. There do, however, seem to be modes of justification which are necessarily truth-indicative. If, as I argued in 4.4, it is necessarily true that the occurrence of (red thing)-type experiences is strong fallible evidence of the presence of red things then necessarily beliefs justifiably formed in response to (red thing)-type experiences, via the type of justification which I called *Q*-justification, would by and large be true.[8] The same would apply to all modes of *Q*-justification since these pertain to types of belief concerning how things appear and rely on what are arguably non-contingent evidential links. Sophisticated sceptics might try to undermine this position (and succeed), but even granted the position it is open to them to claim that for each mode of justification leading to beliefs about the world which 'go beyond' how things presently appear, it is possible that justification in that mode is not genuine because not truth-indicative. It is not clear how this claim could be resisted given the pervasiveness of our reliance on groundless beliefs in contingent evidential links and allied assumptions about live alternatives.

How can the sceptic proceed from here? Notoriously the following inference is not valid.

(i) For every mode of justification *m* pertaining to belief types whose instances go beyond present appearances, it is possible that justification in mode *m* is not genuine.

Therefore,

(ii) it is possible that, for every mode of justification *m* pertaining to belief types whose instances go beyond present appearances, justification in mode *m* is not genuine.

If one thinks that real possibilities must be such that their actualization is in principle detectable then one may be prepared to accept (i) and resist (ii).[9] You can be in a position to discover that a justification in some mode is not genuine only if you have a stable body of background beliefs and beliefs relating to particular cases which go beyond present appearances and are not open to question. In so far as you have these beliefs you are committed to a range of conceptual practices which you could not coherently adopt if you thought that all modes of justification relating to beliefs which go beyond appearances were suspect. Even so, it is not clear that sceptics need argue for (ii). For they can argue that given (i) the *S*-system is compromised so

[8] Compare Wright (1986, 1988).
[9] For a discussion along these lines, see Wright (1986).

far as it concerns beliefs which go beyond appearances, since with regard to each mode of justification relating to such beliefs we have no assurance that justification in that mode is genuine. But now, even beliefs about appearances are justificationally dependent on beliefs which go beyond appearances, for example, beliefs about countervailing facts. So the entire *S*-system is compromised in that our best evaluations of beliefs with respect to justification may as often as not fail to identify beliefs which are genuinely justified. That in itself is scepticism of a radical kind.

This sophisticated sceptical strategy is no doubt open to objection at a number of points, but I shall focus attention on *JUS*(*GEN*). In the next section I shall argue that it is false.

7.4. *A Response to Sophisticated Scepticism*

The sophisticated strategy stems from a conception of the point of evaluating beliefs with respect to justification. According to this conception the point of such evaluations is to assess beliefs in relation to whether holding them is conducive to realizing the aim of believing only what is true. The suggestion is that a belief held on such-and-such grounds will be commendable from this point of view only if holding beliefs on grounds of that sort reliably yields true beliefs. The sophisticated sceptic thinks that the trouble with the *S*-system arises because of the possibility of its containing modes of justification which are not truth-indicative. If your justification for holding some belief is of that type then the grounds on which you hold the belief will not be of a sort which reliably yields true beliefs. In that case, according to the conception just outlined, to hold beliefs on such grounds does not serve the aim of holding only true beliefs.

The key question to consider is what aiming to have only true beliefs requires of us. Certainly it requires us to take such steps as are feasible to ensure that we believe only what is true. But what steps are feasible? Any steps we take proceed from a starting-point which we have not chosen and could not reject wholesale even if we tried. The starting-point is our perspective on the world, which comprises the concepts we have acquired and the propositions which are normative for us (3.2 and 6.3).

Having this perspective commits us to managing our beliefs and evaluating beliefs generally in certain ways. Indeed, if we manage and evaluate beliefs competently it would seem that we do as much as could feasibly be done to serve the aim of believing only what is true. This suggests an alternative conception of the point of evaluating beliefs with respect to justification. The point of such evaluation is not to assess a belief formed on certain grounds in relation to whether forming beliefs on these grounds does in fact more often than not result in true beliefs and thus in fact serves the aim of believing only what is true. The point is rather to assess whether in forming beliefs on these grounds the subject is doing as much as is feasible to serve that aim. If sophisticated sceptics are right we may form a belief competently, on my account, even if the mode of its justification is not truth-indicative. But assuming the alternative conception of the point of evaluating beliefs with respect to justification, the fact that the mode of justification is not truth-indicative would not show that justification in that mode is not genuine. It will be genuine if forming beliefs on the grounds which are implicated in that mode of justification is consistent with doing as much as is feasible to serve the aim of believing only what is true. For all that sophisticated sceptics have argued this may be so.

Doing what is feasible to serve the aim of believing only what is true does not preclude forming beliefs on grounds of a sort which do not reliably yield true beliefs. If grounds of a certain sort are unreliable in this way then forming beliefs on these grounds will not in fact contribute to the aim of believing only what is true. Obviously, if you think that certain grounds are unreliable you should not form beliefs on these grounds. But from where you start and have to start you may have no reason to think this, nor any reason to take the possibility into account in your reasoning.

Why should we prefer the alternative conception of the point of evaluation with respect to justification to that which provides the rationale for *JUS*(*GEN*)? An adequate reason for doing so is that it accords with our evaluative practice. The very fact that we do evaluate beliefs in accordance with the *S*-system shows this to be so. This does not beg the question against sophisticated sceptics. The sophisticated sceptical strategy depends on the idea that *JUS*(*GEN*) reflects our ordinary thinking about justification. This is what enables the sophisticated sceptic to avoid the charge laid against the crude sceptic of imposing conditions of justification which have no proper rationale. But *JUS*(*GEN*) does not in fact accord with our evaluative practice and so the sophisticated strategy is undermined.

Suppose the alternative conception of the point of evaluating beliefs with respect to justification is accepted. It might be suggested by way of an objection to the foregoing line of thought that people who hold *S*-justified beliefs do not always do as much as is feasible to serve the aim of believing only what is true. A radical version of this suggestion would have it that we could be pure enquirers in Bernard Williams's sense, that is, enquirers who set aside all considerations except those internal to enquiry and the search for truth.[10] Then, the argument goes, faced with the sophisticated sceptic's considerations, we would want to check out our groundless beliefs to see if they might be criticized. Why is it not feasible for us to be pure enquirers? Clearly there are practical difficulties. And if part of the project is to suspend beliefs which are not known to pass muster then there would be psychological difficulties too. We cannot suspend all beliefs not known to pass muster. Again, the very idea that we could conduct a global check on our groundless beliefs is incoherent since any checking would require us to take some things for granted which we have not checked.

Still, even if we cannot feasibly be pure enquirers it might be thought that we could feasibly be more assiduous in our enquiries than competence in handling our perspective requires. For instance, when making inferences from strong fallible evidence to a hypothesis *h* could we not take into account at least some alternatives to *h* which we would not ordinarily count as live, but which could for all that provide the true explanation of the evidence? In the deer track case (2.4) could we not check out explicitly whether the tracks have been produced by a crazy track forger? Here I think the difficulty is to see how we can better serve the aim of believing only what is true by enquiring into possibilities which we do not in fact think have any significant chance of being true. It is not just laziness which stops the gamekeeper from reckoning with the

[10] Bernard Williams (1978), ch. 2.

possibility that the tracks are fake. Enquiry on that score would be futile.

The lesson is that we have to make do with the tools at our disposal. These are the concepts and normative propositions of the perspectives which we acquire. But we are not stuck with these come what may. As I have repeatedly stressed throughout we can and should make local adjustments when the need arises.

Thus far I have been concerned with the idea that justifying grounds must be such as reliably to yield true beliefs. But the considerations which are adduced in favour of that view might equally be used to show that we should not hold any beliefs unless on grounds of a sort which reliably yield true beliefs. Holding beliefs on no grounds at all would be ruled out on such a view. The issue here is essentially that raised towards the end of 6.3. How can it be that aiming to believe only what is true generates less than an unqualified grounding requirement? The right response, I think, is akin to that which undermines sophisticated scepticism. In aiming to believe only what is true we cannot feasibly do other than start from where we are, that is, from our perspective. Since that involves having groundless beliefs, having such beliefs cannot be held to be inconsistent with aiming to believe only what is true.

Bibliography

ALBRITTON, ROGERS (1959). 'On Wittgenstein's Use of the Term "Criterion"', *Journal of Philosophy*, 56. Repr. in Pitcher (1968).

ALSTON, WILLIAM P. (1985). 'Concepts of Epistemic Justification', *The Monist*, 68.

ARMSTRONG, D. M. (1963). *Perception and the Physical World* (London: Routledge & Kegan Paul).

—— (1968). *A Materialist Theory of the Mind* (London: Routledge & Kegan Paul).

—— (1973). *Belief, Truth and Knowledge* (Cambridge: Cambridge University Press).

AYER, A. J. (1956). *The Problem of Knowledge* (Harmondsworth: Penguin Books).

AYERS, MICHAEL (1986). 'Are Locke's "Ideas" Images, Intentional Objects or Natural Signs?', *Locke Newsletter*, 17.

BENNETT, JONATHAN (1971). *Locke, Berkeley, Hume: Central Themes* (Oxford: Clarendon Press).

BLACK, MAX (ed.) (1965). *Philosophy in America* (London: Allen & Unwin).

BLACKBURN, SIMON (1973). *Reason and Prediction* (Cambridge: Cambridge University Press).

BLOCK, NED (ed.) (1980). *Readings in the Philosophy of Psychology*, i (Cambridge, Mass.: Harvard University Press).

BOGDAN, RADU J. (ed.) (1986). *Belief: Form, Content and Function* (Oxford: Clarendon Press).

BONJOUR, LAURENCE (1985). *The Structure of Empirical Knowledge* (Cambridge, Mass.: Harvard University Press).

BOWER, TOM (1985). *The Perceptual World of the Child* (London: Fontana Press).

BROWN, STUART C. (ed.) (1977). *Reason and Religion* (Ithaca and London: Cornell University Press).

BRUCE, VICKI, and GREEN, PATRICK (1985). *Visual Perception: Physiology, Psychology and Ecology* (London: Lawrence Erlbaum Associates).

BUCHDAHL, GERD (1969). *Metaphysics and the Philosophy of Science* (Oxford: Blackwell).

BUDD, MALCOLM (1987). 'Wittgenstein on Seeing Aspects', *Mind*, 46.

BURNYEAT, MYLES (1980). 'Can the Skeptic Live his Skepticism?', in Schofield, Burnyeat, and Barnes (1980). Repr. in Burnyeat (1983).

—— (ed.) (1983). *The Skeptical Tradition* (Berkeley: University of California Press).

CAHN, STEVEN M., and SHATZ, DAVID (eds.) (1982). *Contemporary Philosophy of Religion* (New York: Oxford University Press).
CAMPBELL, JOHN (1986). 'Conceptual Structure', in Travis (1986).
CHIHARA, C. S., and FODOR, J. A. (1965). 'Operationalism and Ordinary Language: A Critique of Wittgenstein', *American Philosophical Quarterly*, 2. Repr. in Pitcher (1968).
CHISHOLM, RODERICK M. (1957). *Perceiving: A Philosophical Study* (Ithaca: Cornell University Press).
CHURCHLAND, PAUL M. (1979). *Scientific Realism and the Plasticity of Mind* (Cambridge: Cambridge University Press).
—— (1984). *Matter and Consciousness* (Cambridge, Mass.: MIT Press).
COHEN, L. JONATHAN (1981). 'Can Human Irrationality be Demonstrated?', *Behavioral and Brain Sciences*, 4.
—— (1986). *The Dialogue of Reason* (Oxford: Clarendon Press).
DAVIDSON, DONALD (1983). 'A Coherence Theory of Truth and Knowledge', in Henrich (1983). Repr. in LePore (1986).
—— (1984). *Truth and Interpretation* (Oxford: Clarendon Press).
DENNETT, DANIEL (1969). *Content and Consciousness* (London: Routledge & Kegan Paul).
—— (1982). 'Beyond Belief', in Woodfield (1982).
DUMMETT, MICHAEL (1978). *Truth and Other Enigmas* (London: Duckworth).
—— (1981). *Frege: Philosophy of Language*, 2nd edn. (London: Duckworth).
DURKHEIM, ÉMILE (1976). *The Elementary Forms of the Religious Life*, 2nd edn. (London: Allen & Unwin).
EVANS, GARETH (1982). *The Varieties of Reference* (Oxford: Clarendon Press).
FEIGL, HERBERT, and SCRIVEN, MICHAEL (eds.) (1956). *Minnesota Studies in the Philosophy of Science*, i (Minneapolis: University of Minnesota Press).
FODOR, JERRY (1983). *The Modularity of Mind* (Cambridge, Mass.: MIT Press).
—— (1986). 'Individualism and Supervenience', *Proceedings of the Aristotelian Society*, Suppl. Vol. 60. Repr. with minor revisions in Fodor (1987).
—— (1987). *Psychosemantics* (Cambridge, Mass.: MIT Press).
GEACH, PETER (1957). *Mental Acts* (London: Routledge & Kegan Paul).
GOLDMAN, ALVIN (1976). 'Discrimination and Perceptual Knowledge', *Journal of Philosophy*, 73. Repr. in Pappas and Swain (1978).
—— (1979). 'What is Justified Belief?', in Pappas (1979).
—— (1985). 'The Relation between Epistemology and Psychology', *Synthese*, 64.
—— (1986). *Epistemology and Cognition* (Cambridge, Mass.: Harvard University Press).

GOLDSTEIN, E. BRUCE (1984). *Sensation and Perception*, 2nd edn. (Belmont, Calif.: Wadsworth Publishing Co.).

GOODMAN, NELSON (1965). *Fact, Fiction and Forecast*, 2nd edn. (Indianapolis: Bobbs-Merrill).

GUNDERSON, KEITH (ed.) (1975). *Minnesota Studies in the Philosophy of Science*, vii (Minneapolis: University of Minnesota Press).

GUTTENPLAN, SAMUEL (ed.) (1975). *Mind and Language* (Oxford: Clarendon Press).

HACKER, P. M. S. (1972). *Insight and Illusion* (Oxford: Clarendon Press).

HALDANE, JOHN (1988). 'Understanding Folk', *Proceedings of the Aristotelian Society*, Suppl. Vol. 62.

HAMLYN, D. W. (1983). *Perception, Learning and the Self* (London: Routledge & Kegan Paul).

HANSON, N. R. (1958). *Patterns of Discovery* (Cambridge: Cambridge University Press).

HARMAN, GIBERT (1973). *Thought* (Princeton, NJ: Princeton University Press).

—— (1984). 'Logic and Reasoning', *Synthese*, 60.

—— (1986). *Change in View* (Cambridge, Mass.: MIT Press).

HEIL, JOHN (1983). *Perception and Cognition* (Berkeley and Los Angeles: University of California Press).

HENRICH, D. (ed.) (1983). *Kant oder Hegel* (Stuttgart: Klett-Cotta).

HESSE, MARY (1974). *The Structure of Scientific Inference* (London: Macmillan).

HINTON, J. M. (1973). *Experiences* (Oxford: Clarendon Press).

HOLLIS, MARTIN, and LUKES, STEVEN (eds.) (1982). *Rationality and Relativism* (Oxford: Blackwell).

HONDERICH, TED (ed.) (1985). *Morality and Objectivity* (London: Routledge & Kegan Paul).

HOOKWAY, CHRISTOPHER (1988). *Quine* (Oxford: Polity Press).

HUME, DAVID (1888). *A Treatise of Human Nature*, ed. L. A. Selby-Bigge (Oxford: Clarendon Press).

—— (1902). *An Enquiry Concerning Human Understanding*, ed. L. A. Selby-Bigge, 2nd edn. (Oxford: Clarendon Press).

—— (1970). *Dialogues Concerning Natural Religion*, ed. with a commentary by Nelson Pike (Indianapolis: Bobbs-Merrill).

KANT, IMMANUEL (1933). *Critique of Pure Reason*, trans. by Norman Kemp-Smith, 2nd imp. (London: Macmillan).

KIEFER, H., and MUNITZ, M. (eds.) (1970). *Language, Belief and Metaphysics* (New York: State University of New York Press).

KORNBLITH, HILARY (1980). 'Beyond Foundationalism and the Coherence Theory', *Journal of Philosophy*, 72, repr. in Kornblith (1985).

—— (ed.) (1985). *Naturalizing Epistemology* (Cambridge, Mass.: MIT Press).

LEPORE, ERNEST (ed.) (1986). *Truth and Interpretation* (Oxford: Blackwell).

LEWIS, DAVID (1980). 'Mad Pain and Martian Pain', in Block (1980). Repr. in Lewis (1983).

—— (1983). *Philosophical Papers*, i (Oxford: Oxford University Press).

LOCKE, JOHN (1979). *An Essay Concerning Human Understanding*, ed. Peter H. Nidditch. (Oxford: Clarendon Press).

LUPER-FOY, STEPHEN (1985). 'The Reliabilist Theory of Rational Belief', *The Monist*, 68.

LYCAN, WILLIAM G. (1971). 'Noninductive Evidence: Recent Work on Wittgenstein's "Criteria"', *American Philosophical Quarterly*, 8.

—— (1986). 'Tacit Belief', in Bogdan (1986). Repr. in Lycan (1988).

—— (1988). *Judgement and Justification* (Cambridge: Cambridge University Press).

LYONS, WILLIAM (1986). *The Disappearance of Introspection* (Cambridge, Mass.: MIT Press).

MCDOWELL, JOHN (1982). 'Criteria, Defeasibility and Knowledge', *Proceedings of the British Academy*, 68.

—— (1985). 'Values and Secondary Qualities', in Honderich (1985).

MCGINN, COLIN (1982*a*). 'The Structure of Content', in Woodfield (1982).

—— (1982*b*). *The Character of Mind* (Oxford: Oxford University Press).

—— (1983). *The Subjective View* (Oxford: Clarendon Press).

MALCOLM, NORMAN (1977). 'The Groundlessness of Belief', in Brown (1977).

MILLAR, ALAN (1985*a*). 'Veridicality: More on Searle', *Analysis*, 45.

—— (1985*b*). 'What's in a Look?', *Proceedings of the Aristotelian Society*, New Series, 86.

—— (1989). 'Experience and the Justification of Belief', *Ratio*, 2.

MOORE, G. E. (1959). *Philosophical Papers* (London: Allen & Unwin).

NAGEL, THOMAS (1986). *The View from Nowhere* (New York: Oxford University Press).

NEWTON-SMITH, WILLIAM (1982). 'Relativism and the Possibility of Interpretation', in Hollis and Lukes (1982).

NOZICK, ROBERT (1981). *Philosophical Explanations* (Oxford: Clarendon Press).

O'SHAUGHNESSY, BRIAN (1980). *The Will: A Dual Aspect Theory* (Cambridge: Cambridge University Press).

PAPPAS, GEORGE S. (ed.) (1979). *Justification and Knowledge* (Dordrecht: Reidel).

—— and SWAIN, MARSHALL (eds.) (1978). *Essays on Knowledge and Justification* (Ithaca and London: Cornell University Press).

PASSMORE, JOHN (1968). *Hume's Intentions*, revd. edn. (London: Duckworth).

PEACOCKE, CHRISTOPHER (1979). *Holistic Explanation* (Oxford: Clarendon Press).

—— (1983). *Sense and Content* (Oxford: Clarendon Press).

—— (1986). *Thoughts: An Essay on Content* (Oxford: Blackwell).

PENELHUM, TERENCE (1983). *God and Skepticism* (Dordrecht: Reidel).

PITCHER, GEORGE (ed.) (1968). *Wittgenstein* (London: Macmillan).

—— (1971). *A Theory of Perception* (Princeton, NJ: Princeton University Press).

PITSON, A. E. (1984). 'Basic Seeing', *Philosophy and Phenomenological Research*, 45.

PLANTINGA, ALVIN (1982). 'Rationality and Religious Belief', in Cahn and Shatz (1982).

POLLOCK, JOHN L. (1987). *Contemporary Theories of Knowledge* (London: Hutchinson).

PUTNAM, HILARY (1970). 'Is Semantics Possible?', in Kiefer and Munitz (1970). Repr. in Putnam (1975*b*).

—— (1975*a*). 'The Meaning of "Meaning"', in Gunderson (1975) and Putnam (1975*b*).

—— (1975*b*). *Mind, Language and Reality, Philosophical Papers*, ii (Cambridge: Cambridge University Press).

QUINE, W. V. (1960). *Word and Object* (Cambridge, Mass.: MIT Press).

—— (1961). *From a Logical Point of View*, 2nd edn. (Cambridge, Mass.: Harvard University Press).

—— (1969*a*). 'Epistemology Naturalized', in Quine (1969*b*). Repr. in Kornblith (1985).

—— (1969*b*). *Ontological Relativity and other essays* (New York: Columbia University Press).

—— (1973). *The Roots of Reference* (La Salle, Ill.: Open Court).

—— (1975). 'The Nature of Natural Knowledge', in Guttenplan (1975).

RIPS, L. J. (1988). 'Deduction', in Sternberg and Smith (1988).

ROCK, IRVIN (1983). *The Logic of Perception* (Cambridge, Mass.: MIT Press).

RORTY, RICHARD (1980). *Philosophy and the Mirror of Nature* (Oxford: Blackwell).

RUSSELL, BERTRAND (1926). *Our Knowledge of the External World* (London: Allen & Unwin).

SCHOFIELD, M., BURNYEAT, M., and BARNES, J. (1980). *Doubt and Dogmatism: Studies in Hellenistic Epistemology* (Oxford: Clarendon Press).

SEARLE, JOHN R. (1983). *Intentionality* (Cambridge: Cambridge University Press).

SELLARS, WILFRED (1954). 'Some Reflections on Language Games', *Philosophy of Science*, 21. Repr. in revised form in Sellars (1963).

—— (1956). 'Empiricism and the Philosophy of Mind', in Feigl and Scriven (1956). Repr. in Sellars (1963).

—— (1963). *Science, Perception and Reality* (London: Routledge & Kegan Paul).

SELLARS, WILFRED (1968). *Science and Metaphysics* (London: Routledge & Kegan Paul).

SEXTUS EMPIRICUS (1933). *The Outlines of Empiricism*, trans. by R. G. Bury in the Loeb Classical Library (Cambridge, Mass.: Harvard University Press).

SHOEMAKER, SIDNEY (1963). *Self-Knowledge and Self-Identity* (Ithaca: Cornell University Press).

STERNBERG, ROBERT J., and SMITH, EDWARD E. (eds.) (1988). *The Psychology of Human Thought* (Cambridge: Cambridge University Press).

STICH, STEVEN (1983). *From Folk Psychology to Cognitive Science* (Cambridge, Mass.: MIT Press).

STRAWSON, P. F. (1957). 'Propositions, Concepts, and Logical Truths', *Philosophical Quarterly*, 7. Repr. in Strawson (1971).

—— (1971). *Logico-Linguistic Papers* (London: Methuen).

STROUD, BARRY (1979). 'Inference, Belief, and Understanding', *Mind*, 88.

—— (1984). *The Significance of Philosophical Scepticism* (Oxford: Clarendon Press).

SWAIN, MARSHALL (1981). *Reasons and Knowledge* (Ithaca and London: Cornell University Press).

THOMSON, JUDITH JARVIS (1965). 'Reasons and Reasoning', in Black (1965).

TOULMIN, STEPHEN, and GOODFIELD, JUNE (1963). *The Fabric of the Heavens* (Harmondsworth: Penguin Books).

TRAVIS, CHARLES (1986). *Meaning and Interpretation* (Oxford: Blackwell).

WATKINS, JOHN (1984). *Science and Scepticism* (London: Hutchinson).

WEISKRANZ, L., WARRINGTON, ELIZABETH K., *et al.* (1974). 'Visual Capacity in the Hemianopic Field Following a Restricted Occipital Ablation', *Brain*, 99.

WILLIAMS, BERNARD (1970). 'Deciding to Believe', in Kiefer and Munitz (1970). Repr. in Williams (1973).

—— (1973). *Problems of the Self* (Cambridge: Cambridge University Press).

—— (1978). *Descartes: The Project of Pure Enquiry* (Harmondsworth: Pelican Books).

WILLIAMS, MICHAEL (1977). *Groundless Belief* (Oxford: Blackwell).

WINTERS, BARBARA (1983). 'Inferring', *Philosophical Studies*, 44.

WITTGENSTEIN, LUDWIG (1958). *Philosophical Investigations* (Oxford: Blackwell).

—— (1969). *On Certainty* (Oxford: Blackwell).

WOODFIELD, ANDREW (ed.) (1982). *Thought and Object* (Oxford: Clarendon Press).

WRIGHT, CRISPIN (1980). *Wittgenstein on the Foundations of Mathematics* (London: Duckworth).

—— (1985). 'Facts and Certainty', *Proceedings of the British Academy*, 71.

—— (1986). 'Rule Following, Meaning and Constructivism', in Travis (1986).

—— (1987). *Realism, Meaning and Truth* (Oxford: Blackwell).

—— (1988). 'Moral Values, Projection and Secondary Properties', *Proceedings of the Aristotelian Society*, Suppl. Vol. 62.

Index